Fast Facts

D1277586

Fast Facts:
Bladder Disorders

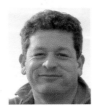

Alex Slack MRCOG
Sub Speciality Trainee in Urogynaecology
Department of Obstetrics and Gynaecology
John Radcliffe Hospital
Oxford, UK

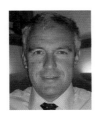

Simon Jackson MA MD FRCOG
Consultant Gynaecologist
Department of Obstetrics and Gynaecology
John Radcliffe Hospital
Oxford, UK

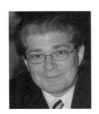

Alan J Wein MD PhD(hon)
Professor and Chair, Division of Urology
University of Pennsylvania School of Medicine
and Health System
Chief of Urology, Hospital of the University of Pennsylvania
Philadelphia, PA, USA

Declaration of Independence
This book is as balanced and as practical as we can make it.
Ideas for improvement are always welcome: feedback@fastfacts.com

HEALTH PRESS

Fast Facts: Bladder Disorders
First published January 2008

Text © 2008 Alex Slack, Simon Jackson, Alan J Wein
© 2008 in this edition Health Press Limited
Health Press Limited, Elizabeth House, Queen Street, Abingdon,
Oxford OX14 3LN, UK
Tel: +44 (0)1235 523233
Fax: +44 (0)1235 523238

Book orders can be placed by telephone or via the website.
For regional distributors or to order via the website, please go to:
www.fastfacts.com
For telephone orders, please call +44 (0)1752 202301 (UK and Europe),
1 800 247 6553 (USA, toll free), +1 419 281 1802 (Americas) or
+61 (0)2 9351 6173 (Asia–Pacific).

Fast Facts is a trademark of Health Press Limited.

All rights reserved. No part of this publication may be reproduced, stored in a
retrieval system, or transmitted in any form or by any means, electronic, mechanical,
photocopying, recording or otherwise, without the express permission of the
publisher.

The rights of Alex Slack, Simon Jackson and Alan J Wein to be identified as the
authors of this work have been asserted in accordance with the Copyright, Designs &
Patents Act 1988 Sections 77 and 78.

The publisher and the authors have made every effort to ensure the accuracy of this
book, but cannot accept responsibility for any errors or omissions.

For all drugs, please consult the product labeling approved in your country for
prescribing information.

Registered names, trademarks, etc. used in this book, even when not marked as such,
are not to be considered unprotected by law.

A CIP record for this title is available from the British Library.

ISBN 978-1-905832-01-9

Slack A (Alex)
Fast Facts: Bladder Disorders/
Alex Slack, Simon Jackson, Alan J Wein

Medical illustrations by Dee McLean, London, UK.
Typesetting and page layout by Zed, Oxford, UK.
Printed by Fine Print (Services) Ltd, Oxford, UK.

Text printed with vegetable inks on biodegradable and
recyclable paper manufactured from sustainable forests.

NORDIC ENVIRONMENTAL LABEL

444   001

Low emissions
during production

Low
chlorine

Sustainable
forests

Glossary 5

Introduction 7

Anatomy and function of the urinary system 9

Assessment 14

Urinary incontinence 31

The overactive bladder 46

Voiding problems 56

Hematuria 64

Urinary tract infections and cystitis 71

Nocturnal symptoms 82

Neuropathic bladder dysfunction 88

Special considerations 94

Useful addresses 105

Index 107

Glossary

ADH: antidiuretic hormone (desmopressin; sometimes abbreviated to DDAVP)

Bacteriuria: presence of bacteria in the urine

BPH: benign prostatic hyperplasia, a major cause of outlet obstruction in men

BTX: botulinum toxin

Compliance: change in bladder volume for a change in intravesical pressure (measured in mL/cmH_2O); bladder compliance is normal if there is little or no change in detrusor pressure during normal filling

CT: computed tomography

Detrusor overactivity: urodynamic observation of involuntary detrusor contraction during bladder filling

DSD: detrusor–sphincter dyssynergia; loss of coordination between detrusor contraction and relaxation of the external urethral sphincter

Dysuria: pain on urination

Fistula: abnormal communication between two epithelialized structures

Frequency: complaint of voiding too often during the day; more than eight voids per 24 hours

Frequency/volume chart: *see* Urinary diary

Glycosuria: presence of glucose in the urine

Hematuria: presence of blood in the urine; may be microscopic or macroscopic/gross (blood evident in the urine)

Hesitancy: difficulty in initiating micturition

IC: interstitial cystitis; may also be referred to as painful bladder syndrome (PBS)

Intermittent stream: urine flow that stops and starts

IVU: intravenous urography

Mixed incontinence: coexistence of stress incontinence with urge incontinence symptoms

NICE: National Institute for Health and Clinical Excellence; the UK organization that provides guidance on health interventions in the UK

Nocturia: complaint of having to void one or more times during the night

Nocturnal enuresis: loss of urine during sleep (bed-wetting)

Nocturnal polyuria: passing more than one-third of the 24-hour output at night

Overactive bladder (OAB): a symptom syndrome that includes urgency (see below), with or without urge urinary incontinence, usually with frequency and nocturia

PBS: painful bladder syndrome

Polyuria: passing of an excessively large volume of urine over a given period

PSA: prostate-specific antigen

Pyuria: presence of pus in the urine

Retention: inability to urinate

Slow stream: reduced urine flow

Stress incontinence: involuntary loss of urine during physical exertion

Terminal dribble: prolonged final part of micturition, when flow slows to a trickle

TVT: tension-free vaginal tape: a suburethral sling that is inserted in a minimally invasive procedure to provide support for the urethra for the treatment of stress incontinence

Urge incontinence: involuntary leakage of urine accompanied by, or immediately preceded by, urgency

Urgency: sudden compelling desire to void that is difficult to defer

Urinary diary: patient-maintained record of fluid intake, and volume and timing of micturition

UTI: urinary tract infection

VVF: vesicovaginal fistula

Introduction

'Bladder disorders' is an inclusive term that encompasses a number of lower urinary tract dysfunctions and abnormalities, which affect a significant number of individuals. These disorders can have a substantial negative effect on quality of life, and some can cause considerable morbidity and even mortality.

This book was written with the non-specialist healthcare professional in mind, to provide the 'fundamentals' related to a number of these disorders – enough to recognize the symptoms and signs, understand the basic pathophysiology and institute initial evaluation and, where appropriate, initial treatment.

We intended the content to be as evidence- and expert-opinion-based as possible, balanced where opinions are not unanimous and, above all, practical. Ideas for improvement are welcome.

1 Anatomy and function of the urinary system

Anatomy

A complete description of the anatomy of the urinary system is beyond the scope of this book and is of limited interest to the general clinician. However, particular aspects of the anatomy and function of the urinary tract are relevant to understanding bladder disorders and should be familiar to anyone working in the field. The relevant anatomy of the urinary system is shown in Figure 1.1.

Function

Continence is maintained by a complex interaction between the bladder, the urethra, the pelvic floor muscles, the endopelvic fascia and the nervous system. The bladder operates as a low-pressure, high-volume system, pressure increasing slowly and steadily as the bladder fills, normally at a rate of 0.5–5 mL/minute.

The bladder can usually hold 500–600 mL urine. A first need to void is felt when the bladder contains 250–300 mL. Continence is maintained as long as the urethral pressure exceeds bladder pressure.

During normal voiding, voluntary relaxation of the striated musculature in and around the urethra precedes contraction of the detrusor muscle. This combination reduces outflow resistance and increases intravesical pressure, causing the bladder to be emptied forcibly.

Urine storage and voiding are controlled by reflex centers in the spinal cord and the micturition center in the midbrain. Both the autonomic and somatic nervous systems are involved. The innervation of the bladder is shown in Figure 1.2. The main neurological pathways that affect bladder contraction are parasympathetic. The sacral reflex center is situated in S2 to S4, and the pelvic nerve and its branches lead from here to the detrusor muscle. Excitation of this nerve stimulates the release primarily of acetylcholine, which acts on muscarinic receptors to cause detrusor contraction.

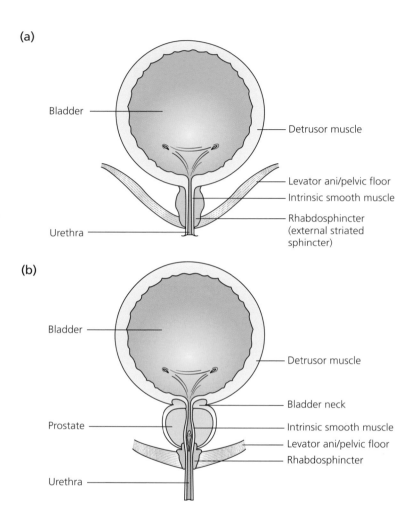

Figure 1.1 Key anatomic features of the (a) female and (b) male urinary systems.

During bladder filling, inhibitory impulses from the micturition center in the brain are transmitted to the sacral micturition center to prevent excitation of the pelvic nerve and suppress detrusor contractions. Voluntary sphincteric innervation is via the pudendal nerve; excitation causes contraction of the external urethral sphincter.

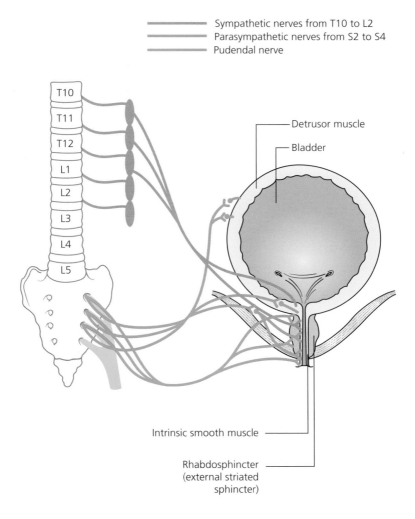

Sympathetic nerves from T10 to L2
Parasympathetic nerves from S2 to S4
Pudendal nerve

T10
T11
T12
L1
L2
L3
L4
L5

Detrusor muscle

Bladder

Intrinsic smooth muscle

Rhabdosphincter
(external striated
sphincter)

Figure 1.2 Innervation of the bladder.

Voiding depends on coordinated excitation of the sacral parasympathetic nerves and simultaneous opening of the bladder outlet (involuntary) and relaxation of the external urethral sphincter (voluntary). Continence requires the converse. The requirements for bladder filling/urine storage and voiding are given in Box 1.1.

BOX 1.1

Requirements for bladder filling/urine storage and voiding

Bladder filling/urine storage requires:

- accommodation of an increasing volume of urine at low intravesical pressure (normal compliance and with normal sensation)
- a bladder outlet that is closed at rest and remains closed during increases in intra-abdominal pressure
- absence of involuntary bladder contractions (detrusor overactivity)

Bladder emptying/voiding requires:

- a coordinated contraction of the bladder smooth musculature of adequate magnitude and duration
- a concomitant lowering of resistance at the level of the smooth and striated sphincter
- absence of anatomic (as opposed to functional) obstruction

Key points – anatomy and function of the urinary system

- The bladder operates as a low-pressure, high-volume system.
- Urine storage and voiding are controlled by reflex centers in the spinal cord, the micturition center in the midbrain and the somatic and parasympathetic nervous systems.
- Voiding requires simultaneous opening of the bladder outlet (involuntary) and relaxation of the external urethral sphincter (voluntary). Continence requires the converse.

Key references

Delancey JO, Ashton-Miller JA.
Pathophysiology of adult urinary
incontinence. *Gastroenterology*
2004;126(1 Suppl 1):S23–32.

Keane DP, O'Sullivan S. Urinary
incontinence: anatomy, physiology
and pathophysiology. *Baillieres Best
Pract Res Clin Obstet Gynaecol*
2000;14:207–26.

Strohbehn K. Normal pelvic floor
anatomy. *Obstet Gynecol Clin North
Am* 1998;25:683–705.

Wein AJ, Moy ML. Voiding
function, dysfunction and urinary
incontinence. In: Hanno P, Wein AJ,
Malkowicz SB, eds. *Penn Clinical
Manual of Urology.* Philadelphia:
Saunders/Elsevier, 2007:341–478.

History

Urologic symptoms are clearly a key aspect in the diagnosis of urinary disorders, but may not be reliable when used alone; as many have stated, the bladder may be an unreliable witness. The onset of urinary symptoms and their duration and severity should be recorded. Symptoms can be divided into filling, storage and voiding/emptying symptoms.

Filling symptoms

Frequency is the complaint of voiding too often by day and can be defined as more than eight voids per 24 hours. Increased daytime frequency can occur with a normal bladder where there is excessive fluid intake, or where the bladder capacity is restricted by detrusor overactivity, impaired bladder compliance (bladder compliance is normal if there is little or no change in detrusor pressure during normal filling) or increased bladder sensation (hypersensitivity). The causes of daytime frequency are shown in Table 2.1.

TABLE 2.1

Causes of daytime urinary frequency

- Detrusor overactivity (urodynamic finding)
- Impaired bladder compliance (urodynamic finding)
- Increased bladder sensation
- Overactive bladder (symptom syndrome)
- Excessive fluid intake
- Diuretic medication
- Diabetes mellitus
- Caffeine (in susceptible individuals)
- Prophylactic voiding (to avoid urgency or urge incontinence)

Nocturia is the complaint of having to void one or more times during the night. It may occur for the same reasons as daytime frequency, but may also occur in association with congestive heart failure or because the normal circadian rhythm of antidiuretic hormone (ADH; desmopressin) secretion becomes reversed.

Urgency is a sudden compelling desire to void that is difficult to defer. Urgency implies detrusor overactivity, but can also occur if there is an underlying bladder inflammatory disorder.

Storage symptoms

Stress (or effort-related) incontinence is the involuntary loss of urine during physical exertion. This occurs without any contraction of the detrusor and may be associated with a number of activities, including coughing, sneezing, running, jumping, aerobics and sexual activity. It is caused by failure of the bladder outlet to remain closed and thereby maintain continence when intra-abdominal pressure is raised.

Urge incontinence is the involuntary leakage of urine accompanied, or immediately preceded, by urgency. Urge incontinence can take the form of frequent small losses between voids or sudden complete bladder emptying. It is caused by involuntary detrusor contractions during bladder filling/urine storage.

Nocturnal enuresis is the loss of urine during sleep. When taking a history, it is important to inquire about childhood nocturnal enuresis, as delayed bladder control in childhood is often associated with detrusor overactivity in adulthood.

Continuous incontinence tends to be associated with urinary tract fistulas or with chronic retention with so-called overflow incontinence. Urinary tract fistulas are usually iatrogenic in developed countries, but are commonly associated with unsupervised childbirth in developing countries. Chronic retention is most common in men with obstruction secondary to prostate enlargement.

Mixed incontinence is the coexistence of stress incontinence with urge incontinence or urge symptoms.

Voiding/emptying symptoms. With the exception of postmicturition dribble, all of the symptoms described below can be associated with bladder outlet obstruction, a poorly contracting detrusor or loss of coordination between detrusor contractility and relaxation of the external urethral sphincter, termed detrusor–sphincter dyssynergia (DSD).

Hesitancy is described as difficulty in initiating micturition, resulting in a delay in the onset of voiding when the individual is ready to pass urine.

Intermittent stream describes urine flow that stops and starts once or more during micturition.

Slow stream is the perception of a reduced urine flow, usually compared with previous performance or with the flow of others.

Terminal dribble describes a prolonged final part of micturition, when the flow slows to a trickle.

Incomplete emptying is a self-explanatory term for a feeling experienced by an individual after passing urine.

Postmicturition dribble refers to the leakage of urine after micturition. Approximately 80% of men experience this symptom at some time and it can present at any age. The symptom arises from the leakage of a few drops of urine that are pooled in the bulbar urethra after micturition has been completed and that drain under gravity a few moments later. Postmicturition dribble is seldom associated with clinical abnormalities, and can be avoided by waiting until the remaining urine has been passed or by milking the urethra at the end of micturition. Urethral stricture or diverticulum may be rare causes of this condition. If voiding dysfunction is present, uroflowmetry should be the first investigation (see page 24).

Physical examination

All patients presenting with bladder symptoms should undergo a full physical examination, including neurological examination.

Neurological examination. Neurological conditions that are associated with bladder problems (such as multiple sclerosis, Parkinson's disease or spinal injury) are usually obvious when the patient first presents.

If a neurological cause is suspected, it is important to pay particular attention to sacral neuronal pathways. The gait, abduction and dorsiflexion of the toes (S3) should be assessed, as should sensory innervation of the perineum (L1–L2), sole and lateral aspect of the foot (S1) and posterior aspect of the thigh (S2). Perineal (S3) and cutaneous reflexes (bulbocavernosus and anal reflexes) should also be tested.

Abdominal examination. Scars from previous surgery should be noted. Increased abdominal striae may be found in association with other markers of abnormal collagen metabolism, and are more common in women with prolapse and stress incontinence.

An attempt to palpate the kidneys should be made. Abdominal examination or suprapubic percussion may identify a distended bladder or a pelvic mass that is compressing the bladder.

Genital examination is essential in both women and men.

Women. The skin of the vulva and perineum should be examined, and any atrophic vaginitis identified. Speculum examination will enable assessment of the vaginal walls to identify atrophy, cystocele, rectocele or uterine or vault prolapse. Pelvic masses may also be identified.

The woman should be asked to cough and strain in an attempt to demonstrate stress incontinence. It may be necessary to examine the woman whilst she stands with one foot on a stool, in order to detect prolapse or stress incontinence.

The strength of the pelvic floor muscles should be assessed and can be quantified using a validated grading system such as the Oxford 1–5 scale. Factors to be assessed include strength, duration and repeatability of contractions, and displacement of the pelvic floor.

Men. The appearance of the external urethral meatus and prepuce may be a guide to distal urethral causes of voiding difficulties or postmicturition dribble that the patient may describe as urinary incontinence (i.e. strictures).

Digital rectal examination (see Figure 5.1, page 59) should include palpation of the prostate to assess size, symmetry and consistency of the gland, its position in relation to the rectum and pelvic side wall and the presence of nodularity or induration. Symptoms of bladder overactivity can be caused by locally advanced prostate cancer. Rectal masses are obviously abnormal and require prompt referral. The status of the anal sphincter musculature should be noted.

Further investigations

Further investigation is usually necessary to confirm the cause of bladder symptoms. The investigations undertaken will depend to some extent on the facilities available.

Psychological examination. A mini mental-state examination can be used to assess an agitated or depressed patient, as incontinence can have behavioral causes. Clinical depression will compromise the success of surgical treatment for stress incontinence.

Quality of life. There are a number of ways to assess the impact of incontinence symptoms on a patient's quality of life. However, the only valid way to measure the patient's perception of their symptoms is through the use of psychometrically robust self-completion questionnaires, such as the international consultation on incontinence modular questionnaire (ICIQ; Figure 2.1) A wide variety of questionnaires were assessed at the third international consultation on incontinence; the questionnaires recommended for the assessment of quality of life for patients with urinary incontinence alone or in the presence of lower urinary tract symptoms are listed in Table 2.2.

TABLE 2.2

Questionnaires recommended by the International Continence Society for assessing quality of life in patients with urinary incontinence

Men and women	International consultation on incontinence modular questionnaire (ICIQ-UI short form; see Figure 2.1)
Women	ICIQ-FLUTS, formerly known as the Bristol female lower urinary tract symptoms short-form questionnaire
	Stress and urge incontinence quality-of-life questionnaire (SUIQQ)
Men	ICIQ-MLUTS, formerly known as the International Continence Society male short-form questionnaire

ICIQ-UI Short Form

Initial number [ ][ ][ ][ ][ ][ ][ ]

CONFIDENTIAL

[ ][ ] [ ][ ] [ ][ ]
DAY   MONTH   YEAR
Today's date

Many people leak urine some of the time. We are trying to find out how many people leak urine, and how much this bothers them. We would be grateful if you could answer the following questions, thinking about how you have been, on average, over the PAST FOUR WEEKS.

1 Please write in your date of birth:

[ ][ ] [ ][ ] [ ][ ]
DAY   MONTH   YEAR

2 Are you *(tick one)*:   Female [ ]   Male [ ]

3 How often do you leak urine? *(Tick one box)*

never	[ ]	0
about once a week or less often	[ ]	1
two or three times a week	[ ]	2
about once a day	[ ]	3
several times a day	[ ]	4
all the time	[ ]	5

4 We would like to know how much urine you think leaks.
How much urine do you usually leak (whether you wear protection or not)?
(Tick one box)

none	[ ]	0
a small amount	[ ]	2
a moderate amount	[ ]	4
a large amount	[ ]	6

5 Overall, how much does leaking urine interfere with your everyday life?
Please ring a number between 0 (not at all) and 10 (a great deal)

0 1 2 3 4 5 6 7 8 9 **10**
not at all   a great deal

ICIQ score: sum scores 3+4+5 [ ] [ ]

6 When does urine leak? *(Please tick all that apply to you)*

never – urine does not leak	[ ]
leaks before you can get to the toilet	[ ]
leaks when you cough or sneeze	[ ]
leaks when you are asleep	[ ]
leaks when you are physically active/exercising	[ ]
leaks when you have finished urinating and are dressed	[ ]
leaks for no obvious reason	[ ]
leaks all the time	[ ]

Thank you very much for answering these questions.

Copyright © "ICIQ Group"

Figure 2.1 This short-form international consultation on incontinence modular questionnaire (ICIQ) is one of a number of questionnaires that have been validated to assess a patient's perception of their symptoms. Reproduced with permission of the ICIQ Group. See www.iciq.net for further information.

Frequency/volume chart. Use of a urinary diary is a simple and practical method to obtain information on a patient's normal voiding pattern, including frequency of micturition and episodes of leakage, in addition to the time and volume of fluid ingested. The patient records the times and volumes of all voids over a specific time period, which should be at least 24 hours so that both day and night are included. Episodes of urinary incontinence are recorded and whether they are associated with urgency, straining, coughing etc. The patient also records fluid intake.

Objective information is obtained not only on daytime frequency and nocturia, but also on the normal functional bladder capacity, mean voided volume, total voided volumes and diurnal distribution of micturition. Abnormalities that may be demonstrated on a frequency/volume chart include:

- regular voiding of small quantities of urine, which is associated with filling abnormalities
- nocturia and nocturnal polyuria (passing more than one-third of the 24-hour output during sleeping hours)
- fluid restriction
- excessive fluid intake (through habit or on medical advice)
- polyuria (an excessive volume of urination, which in an adult would be more than 2500 mL/day)
- urinary incontinence and the associated circumstances (i.e. urgency, effort, unaware).

The frequency/volume chart is also useful for assessing and monitoring treatment, and to demonstrate the benefits of treatment to a patient. Some examples of completed urinary diaries are shown in Figure 2.2.

Urinalysis and culture. Dipstick urinalysis is used to detect hematuria, glycosuria, pyuria and bacteriuria. It should be carried out for all patients presenting with urinary incontinence to exclude the possibility of infection, inflammation, urinary tract malignancy and diabetes. A positive dipstick test should be followed up by formal urine microscopy and culture to detect a urinary tract infection (UTI) before treatment and to allow antibiotic sensitivity to be evaluated. The presence of hematuria or red blood cells on microscopy should be investigated further with urine cytology, an imaging study of the upper tracts

(a)

Time	Intake (mL)	Urine (mL)	Leak
01:00			
02:00			
03:00		150	
04:00			
05:00			
06:00		150	
07:00	250		
08:00		100	
09:00	500		
10:00		100	
11:00	200		
12:00			X
13:00	250	75	
14:00		75	
15:00			
16:00	250	100	
17:00			
18:00			
19:00	500	150	
20:00			
21:00	250	100	
22:00			
23:00			
24:00			

(b)

Time	Intake (mL)	Urine (mL)	Leak
01:00			
02:00			
03:00		200	
04:00			
05:00		200	
06:00			
07:00			
08:00	500	300	
09:00			
10:00			
11:00	250		
12:00			
13:00	300	300	
14:00			
15:00	250		
16:00			
17:00	300	200	
18:00			
19:00			
20:00	300		
21:00			
22:00		200	
23:00			
24:00		250	

Figure 2.2 The frequency/volume chart (urinary diary) is a simple method of highlighting abnormal fluid intake and increased frequency of micturition. The diaries above show (a) regular voiding of small volumes of urine, indicative of a filling disorder; (b) more than one-third of the 24-hour urine output being passed during sleeping hours, indicative of nocturnal polyuria.

(kidneys and ureters) and endoscopic examination of the bladder and urethra to rule out malignancy, especially in a patient over 50 years of age with symptoms of bladder irritation. The investigation and management of hematuria are described in detail in Chapter 6.

Imaging

Radiography. A preliminary plain abdominal radiograph can be performed in patients with suspected renal tract calculi or soft tissue masses.

Ultrasonography has become the first-line method for detecting abnormalities of the kidneys, including scarring, calculi, dilatation and tumors. Ultrasound can also be used to detect increased bladder-wall thickness (which suggests outlet obstruction and/or detrusor overactivity), to look for bladder calculi and to measure postvoid urine volumes.

Intravenous urography has largely been superseded by ultrasonography for initial investigation of microscopic hematuria but may be appropriate if ultrasonography suggests obstruction or leakage from a fistula.

Computed tomography (CT) urography has become the investigation of choice if ultrasonography is not diagnostic or gross hematuria is present. It has a higher sensitivity for small calculi and early neoplasms.

Urodynamic studies

These include methods that generate quantitative data relevant to events in the bladder and bladder outlet during the filling/storage and emptying/voiding phases of miturition.

Many clinicians request urodynamic investigation for any patient, especially a woman, who complains of lower urinary tract symptoms; however, the clinician may have little appreciation of the clinical indications, what the test involves and its limitations. Urodynamic investigation is safe, but men in particular will experience some discomfort related to catheterization, which can last for up to 24 hours after the test. The incidence of culture-proven UTI following urodynamic testing is approximately 1%; prophylactic antibiotics should therefore be considered for patients who may be at risk.

Indications. Urodynamic investigation may be indicated in the following cases:

- treatment failure
- complex mixed lower urinary tract symptoms
- before incontinence surgery
- symptoms suggesting detrusor overactivity
- voiding symptoms
- neuropathic bladder.

Complex mixed lower urinary tract symptoms or treatment failure. Some patients present with such a complicated history that it is impossible to make any judgment as to the cause of their symptoms. Empirical treatment is therefore not possible. The patient should undergo urodynamic investigation so that appropriate treatment can be offered.

Before incontinence surgery. In our opinion, urodynamic information is essential if surgery to treat incontinence, especially stress incontinence, is contemplated. There is, however, some debate as to the need for urodynamic investigation before incontinence surgery. The UK's National Institute for Health and Clinical Excellence (NICE) has recently issued guidelines stating that preoperative urodynamic studies are not necessary for patients undergoing a primary procedure and whose symptoms and examination findings suggest simple stress incontinence. We disagree with this recommendation, as it has been claimed that surgery carried out on the basis of symptoms is inappropriate in 25% of cases. Furthermore, surgery for stress incontinence can lead to voiding dysfunction and de novo detrusor overactivity, or may exacerbate pre-existing symptoms, so it is important to perform a preoperative assessment.

Symptoms suggesting detrusor overactivity. Most patients with symptoms suggestive of detrusor overactivity can be treated empirically. Urodynamic investigation is appropriate if symptoms of detrusor overactivity are unresponsive to drug therapy and if the diagnosis is essential, either to avoid unnecessary continuation of drugs or to exclude other pathology. It is important to understand that urodynamic study provides only an artificial 10–20 minute 'snapshot' and does not always replicate real-life events. Thus, a patient with symptoms of detrusor overactivity may have a normal urodynamic study. Some of

23

these patients will have detrusor overactivity that has been missed, and a trial of therapy is entirely appropriate.

Voiding symptoms are more common in men than women, reflecting a higher incidence of bladder outlet obstruction; however, voiding symptoms do occur in women, especially in association with prolapse or poor detrusor contractility. The initial investigation should be measurement of free urinary flow and postvoid residual volume. If abnormal emptying is confirmed, full urodynamic assessment is required to differentiate between detrusor hypocontractility and outlet obstruction.

Neuropathic bladder. Patients with neurological disease and lower urinary tract symptoms are at risk of neurogenic detrusor overactivity, low compliance and DSD. The main concern is the potential for upper urinary tract damage resulting from raised detrusor/intravesical pressure, which can lead to ureteric dilatation and renal impairment. A simultaneous investigation of the renal tract anatomy and function is essential in these patients (videocystourethrography with concurrent urodynamic investigation).

Uroflowmetry is a simple test in which the patient voids in privacy into a commode that incorporates a urinary flowmeter, measuring urine flow over time (Figure 2.3). A voided volume of at least 150–200 mL is necessary for the flow rate to be interpreted accurately. A normal finding consists of:

- total voided volume greater than 200 mL
- volume passed over a period of 15–20 seconds
- maximum flow rate above 20 mL/second
- smooth crescendo parabolic curve.

It should be recognized that most 'normal' data relate to flowmetry in patients younger than 55 years of age; thus, flow rate should be interpreted with consideration for the minimum acceptable flow for given sex and age groups.

Subsequent measurement of the postvoid residual volume by bladder scanning or catheterization gives further information about bladder emptying.

Cystometry records bladder pressure during filling and voiding, with the aim of explaining a clinical problem in pathophysiological terms. The bladder is filled with saline at room temperature via a small-bore urethral catheter, alongside which is passed a fine pressure transducer. The pressure in the rectum is recorded simultaneously to differentiate rises in intravesical pressure secondary to increases in abdominal

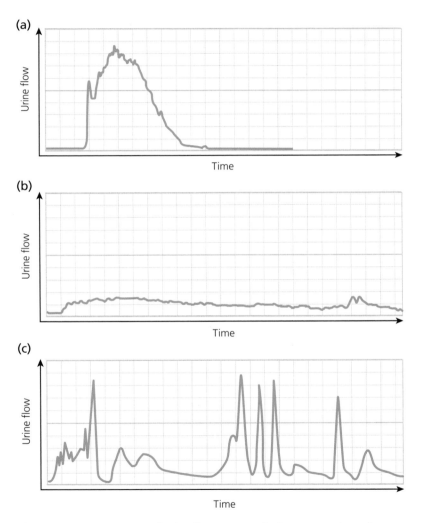

Figure 2.3 Measurement of urine flow rate can indicate a number of abnormalities. (a) Normal voiding. (b) Reduced flow in a man with prostate outlet obstruction. (c) Intermittent increases in flow in a patient straining to void.

pressure (e.g. coughing, straining, talking and changing position) from those due to detrusor contractions. Table 2.3 lists the measurements required during filling cystometry. Figure 2.4 shows some typical traces.

Filling cystometry is unphysiological in that the bladder is normally filled at a very slow rate without any change in pressure, and higher filling rates may produce significant artifacts, particularly in patients with neurological problems. Filling rates are classified as follows:

- fast: above 100 mL/minute
- medium: 10–100 mL/min
- slow: less than 10 mL/min.

A filling rate of 50–60 mL/min during conventional filling cystometry appears to be a good compromise, allowing practical filling times with a low incidence of artifacts.

The following can be evaluated during filling cystometry.

- Capacity – the volume infused during filling is measured, and hence the bladder volume is calculated.
- Sensation – the patient is asked to comment on bladder sensation during filling.
- First sensation of bladder filling – this is the feeling that the patient has when he or she first becomes aware of bladder filling during filling cystometry, usually at about half capacity (150–200 mL).
- First desire to void – this is the feeling that leads the patient to pass urine at the next convenient moment, although voiding can be delayed if necessary; commonly at 75% of capacity.

TABLE 2.3

Measurements required during filling cystometry

Intravesical pressure	Usually measured manometrically with a fluid-filled urethral catheter
Intra-abdominal pressure	Measured manometrically with a fluid-filled rectal catheter
Detrusor pressure	Total intravesical pressure minus intra-abdominal pressure
Volume infused	Equates to the bladder volume
Urine flow rate	Measured by mechanical flowmeter

- Strong desire to void – this is a persistent desire to void but without fear of leakage, felt at capacity.
- Urgency – this is a sudden compelling desire to void, described particularly by patients with detrusor overactivity or inflammatory bladder conditions.

(a)

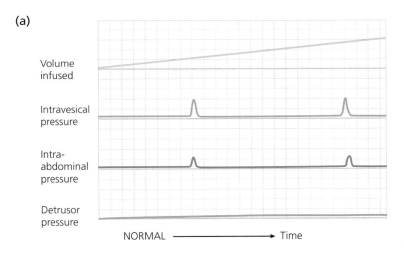

NORMAL ⟶ Time

(b)

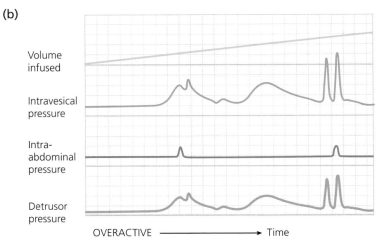

OVERACTIVE ⟶ Time

Figure 2.4 Examples of traces obtained from cystometry. (a) A normal trace. (b) Detrusor overactivity. The terms are described in Table 2.3.

- Maximum cystometric capacity – this is the volume at which the patient feels unable to delay micturition. (The test is usually stopped before this.)
- Detrusor function – abnormal detrusor contractions during bladder filling are noted; detrusor contractility during voiding can be assessed by recording the detrusor pressure in the voiding phase.
- Compliance – this indicates the change in volume for a change in pressure and is expressed in mL/cmH_2O. Little or no pressure change occurs during normal filling in a patient with normal compliance. Compliance may be reduced if bladder pathology is present.
- Urethral function – an incompetent urethral closure mechanism is defined as one that allows leakage of urine in the absence of a detrusor contraction. Stress incontinence can be demonstrated by asking the patient to cough during the filling phase. If urine loss is noted, the subtracted detrusor pressure trace should be checked to ensure that there is no associated detrusor contraction. If stress incontinence has not been demonstrated once the functional bladder capacity is reached, the filling catheter can be removed, leaving a pressure-recording catheter or transducer in place, and the patient asked to undertake a variety of provocative maneuvers, such as coughing, squatting, heel bouncing and jumping.

Voiding cystometry (pressure–flow study). When filling cystometry has been completed, the filling line is removed as described above, and the patient is asked to void with the bladder and abdominal pressure transducers still in place. The urinary flow rate and detrusor pressure are recorded. A normal man voids with a detrusor pressure of $20–40$ cmH_2O and a normal woman with a considerably lower pressure of $0–25$ cmH_2O. Measurement of detrusor pressure gives an indication of the contractility of the bladder and, when combined with the urinary flow rate, the outflow resistance: high pressures and low flow rates indicate outlet obstruction.

Videourodynamic investigation combines cystometry with simultaneous radiological screening of the bladder and urethra. A radiopaque contrast medium is used instead of saline. Videourodynamic investigation provides information about the appearance of the bladder, urethra and sphincters, and will identify reflux into the ureters. It may be more useful than cystometry alone in the assessment of complex cases. It is especially useful to identify the site of obstruction in an individual with high pressure–low flow and to differentiate low pressure–low flow from outlet obstruction.

Ambulatory urodynamic investigation. In complex cases, the artifact created by fast filling can be removed by using natural-fill cystometry and long-term ambulatory urodynamic investigations. This technique involves using microtip pressure transducers to record rectal and bladder pressures. The signals are digitized and stored in the memory of the device. If the machine incorporates an integrated voiding channel, data from a flowmeter can also be stored. First desire to void, urgency, micturition and subjective leaking can then be recorded in the memory using event marker buttons. Studies can last for up to 24–48 hours depending on the memory available. Urine loss can be measured objectively by recording the increase in pad weight during the test.

Ambulatory urodynamic investigations are useful in patients who have incontinence not seen on conventional urodynamics. Recording over two or three natural filling–voiding cycles allows correlation between the patient's symptoms, the detrusor pressure and episodes of incontinence.

Diagnostic cystourethroscopy can be carried out using either a rigid or a flexible cystoscope, with or without anesthesia. Water is the preferred distension medium used during cystoscopy. An angled cystoscope (30 or 70 degrees) is normally required to visualize the whole of the bladder. Comment should be made on the appearance of the urethra, trigone, bladder mucosa and ureteric orifices. If bladder filling symptoms are present, the volume of fluid infused should be noted.

Diagnostic cystourethroscopy is indicated in cases of recurrent UTI, hematuria, bladder pain and suspected bladder injury. It is also used intraoperatively when carrying out continence procedures and when inserting suprapubic catheters.

Key points – assessment

- Urologic symptoms are key in the diagnosis of urinary disorders: onset, duration and severity should be recorded.
- Urinary symptoms can relate to filling (frequency, nocturia, urgency), storage (stress incontinence, urge incontinence, nocturnal enuresis) or voiding/emptying (hesitancy, intermittent stream, slow stream, terminal dribble, incomplete emptying).
- Physical examination is essential, and may include neurological examination, abdominal examination and examination of the genitals.
- Psychological examination can identify behavioral causes of incontinence; the effect of symptoms on quality of life can be assessed using self-completion questionnaires.
- A frequency/volume chart (urinary diary) is a simple and practical method to record voiding and fluid intake.
- Dipstick urinalysis is essential for all patients with urinary incontinence. Positive tests should be evaluated further.
- Urodynamic investigation can provide a wide variety of information, but is not necessarily indicated for all patients.

Key references

Abrams P, Cardozo L, Fall M et al. The standardisation of terminology in lower urinary tract function: report from the standardization sub-committee of the International Continence Society. *Urology* 2003; 61:37–49.

Martin JL, Williams KS, Abrams KR et al. Systematic review and evaluation of methods of assessing urinary incontinence. *Health Technol Assess* 2006;10:1–132,iii–iv.

McLellan A, Cardozo L. Urodynamic techniques. *Int Urogynecol J Pelvic Floor Dysfunct* 2001;12:266–70.

Rovner ES, Wein AJ. Evaluation of lower urinary tract symptoms in females. *Curr Opin Urol* 2003; 13:273–8.

Definitions

Urinary incontinence (UI) is defined as the involuntary loss of urine. A classification of UI is given in Table 3.1. Stress incontinence, which is the focus of this chapter, is defined as the involuntary leakage of urine

---

TABLE 3.1

Classification of urinary incontinence

Extraurethral

- Fistula (vesico-, uretero-, urethrovaginal)
- Ectopic urethra

Urethral

Functional

- Due to physical disability
- Due to lack of awareness or concern

Postvoid dribbling

- Urethral diverticulum
- Vaginal pooling of blood

Outlet underactivity

- 'Genuine' stress urinary incontinence
    - Lack of urethral support
    - Hypermobility, deficient 'hammock'
- Intrinsic sphincter deficiency
    - Neurological disease/injury
    - Fibrosis
- Urethral instability

Bladder overactivity

- Involuntary contractions
    - Neurological disease/injury
    - Bladder outlet obstruction
    - Afferent activation (including inflammation/infection)
    - Idiopathic
- Decreased compliance
    - Neurological disease/injury
    - Fibrosis
    - Idiopathic
- Combination of the above

'Overflow' incontinence

Adapted from Wein and Moy 2007.

on effort or exertion. Urge incontinence is the involuntary leakage of urine accompanied, or immediately preceded, by urgency, and is largely caused by involuntary detrusor contractions during bladder filling/storage. This is discussed in more detail in Chapter 4. Mixed incontinence refers to the coexistence of stress incontinence with urge incontinence symptoms.

Epidemiology

The prevalence of UI in women is difficult to estimate, and differs according to the setting studied. In the general population, estimates vary from 5% among women aged 15 years and older in Belgium, to 69% among women aged 19 years and older in Wales. Most estimates are in the range of 25–45%. The prevalence of UI increases up to about 50 years of age, then levels off until 70 years of age before starting to rise again. The type of incontinence also varies with age. In surveys of older women, mixed and urge incontinence predominate, whereas stress incontinence is generally the dominant symptom in young and middle-aged women.

The prevalence of UI in men has been reported to range from 3% to 39%, and it is generally agreed that the prevalence is less than half that in women. Urge incontinence predominates (40–80%), followed by mixed urinary incontinence (10–30%) and stress urinary incontinence (less than 10%).

In general, the prevalence of UI in nursing-home residents is about 50% in both sexes.

Quality of life

UI has a major impact on quality of life, measured using both general and specific questionnaires (see pages 18–19). UI primarily affects self-esteem, ability to maintain an independent lifestyle, social interactions with friends and family, activities of daily life, and sexual activity.

Risk factors for urinary incontinence

There are situations in which urinary incontinence cannot be considered merely as an isolated abnormality of either bladder contractility or sphincter resistance. These situations, listed in Table 3.2, are

TABLE 3.2

Combined problems associated with incontinence

- Detrusor overactivity with outlet obstruction
- Detrusor overactivity with impaired bladder contractility
- Sphincteric incontinence with impaired bladder contractility
- Sphincteric incontinence with detrusor overactivity

Adapted from Wein & Moy 2007.

complicated to deal with because, first, they are difficult to diagnose, and, second, one entity may adversely affect or compromise treatment of the other.

Stress incontinence

Stress incontinence is the involuntary leakage of urine on effort, exertion, sneezing or coughing, and suggests a problem with the bladder outlet. Urodynamic stress incontinence is noted during filling cystometry and is defined as the involuntary leakage of urine during increased abdominal pressure, in the absence of a detrusor contraction.

Women

Obstetric factors can contribute to the development of UI. The effects of pregnancy and delivery on urinary function are discussed in more detail in Chapter 10 (see pages 97–100).

Pregnancy. UI is common during pregnancy and usually resolves in the postpartum period. However, it has been shown to be a predictor for postpartum incontinence, as well as a risk factor for incontinence 5 years after delivery.

Delivery. There is growing evidence that vaginal delivery may predispose women to incontinence. Vaginal delivery has been shown to cause pelvic neuropathy, and other factors may include avulsion injuries to the pelvic ligaments. Studies into the mode of delivery have generally shown that, compared with nulliparous women, the risk of incontinence increases progressively with cesarean section, vaginal delivery and forceps delivery. There is also a suggestion that higher birth weights may predispose the mother to incontinence, the risk increasing with birth weights above 4 kg.

Menopause and reproductive hormones. While it has long been considered that reduction in estrogen levels at the menopause causes atrophic changes that can lead to urinary symptoms, the literature is inconsistent in describing the role of the menopause and estrogen loss as significant contributors to UI. There is no convincing evidence for a role of hormone replacement therapy in the management of incontinence.

Obesity is well established as a factor that contributes to the incidence of UI. It is believed that excessive weight has similar effects to pregnancy, causing chronic strain, stretching and weakening of the pelvic floor muscles and nerves.

Men. Risk factors for urinary stress incontinence in men include age, neurological disease, urinary infection, outlet obstruction, functional and cognitive impairment, and prostatectomy.

Prostatectomy is a well-known cause of incontinence in men. The incidence of stress incontinence following transurethral resection of the prostate is about 1% and is 5–15% after radical prostatectomy.

Diagnosis and assessment

Diagnosis is largely as described in Chapter 2. A detailed clinical history is crucial in any patient with stress UI in order to obtain an accurate diagnosis, and should include assessment of filling and storage symptoms as described in Chapter 2. Physical examination is also important, but neurological examination is rarely relevant, as most neurological abnormalities will be obvious when a patient first presents.

Further investigations may be necessary to elucidate the cause of stress UI; the investigations carried out will to some extent depend on the facilities available and can include frequency/volume charts and dipstick urinalysis. Urodynamic assessment is appropriate for all patients in whom surgical treatment is being considered and in patients with complex symptoms that do not respond to simple conservative measures or drug treatments.

Management of stress incontinence in women

Treatment should initially be conservative and can be implemented without recourse to urodynamic assessment.

Lifestyle. Encouraging weight reduction and smoking cessation (largely to reduce cough), treating chronic cough conditions, and rectifying exacerbating conditions such as constipation can all help in the management of incontinence.

Reduction in caffeine intake decreases incontinence episodes and helps with other conservative measures.

Pelvic floor exercises. The pelvic floor supports the bladder neck, rectum and vagina (Figure 3.1). Exercises to strengthen the pelvic floor, and therefore the bladder neck, were first described by Kegel in 1948. The aims are to promote patient awareness and to improve the contractility and coordination of pelvic floor muscles, especially in women with poor pelvic floor strength.

Exercise regimens concentrate on both contraction strength and muscle endurance. The exercises described in Box 3.1 are best taught by a physiotherapist. A vaginal assessment should be performed to ensure correct technique. Improvement should be observed within 3–4 months.

Physiotherapists employ additional techniques to maximize pelvic floor contractility.

Biofeedback training, which uses a device to convert the effect of pelvic floor contraction into a visual or auditory response, allows patients and health professionals to observe improvement in an objective manner. One such device is a perineometer, which is placed within the vagina and gives a numerical value for the contractile strength of the pelvic floor. However, it will also register raised vaginal pressure secondary to a valsalva maneuver and so cannot be used in isolation.

Pudendal nerve stimulation with an electrode can be useful if the initial pelvic floor contraction is weak. A woman can use the device for 20 minutes a day at home and adjust the strength of stimulation herself.

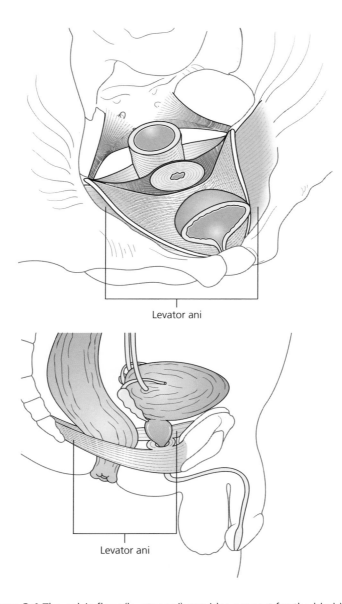

Levator ani

Levator ani

Figure 3.1 The pelvic floor (levator ani) provides support for the bladder neck, vagina and rectum. Weakness in the muscle can contribute to stress incontinence.

BOX 3.1

Instructions: how to perform pelvic floor exercises

- Sit in a comfortable position with your knees slightly apart.
- Imagine that you are trying to stop yourself from passing wind and/or trying to stop the flow of urine.
- You should be aware of a tightening sensation around the back passage and vagina as well as drawing up of the skin away from the crutch of your underwear.
- You should not move your buttocks and thighs at all.
- The muscles need to be tightened firmly and held steadily for up to 10 seconds. In the initial period you may only be able to do this for a few seconds.
- Contractions need to be repeated at least 8–10 times, giving a 5–10 second period of recovery between each repetition.
- In addition to these long contractions it is often advised to perform a series of fast, strong contractions held for only 1–2 seconds.
- Exercises should only take a few minutes and should be performed several times a day.

Weighted vaginal cones can help women to identify the muscles of the pelvic floor (Figure 3.2). Cones of increasing weight (20–90 g) are inserted into the vagina and the woman trains her muscles to prevent the cone from falling out. These cones have proved popular since they were introduced in 1980; subjective improvement rates can be as high as 70%.

Pharmacological treatment

Duloxetine hydrochloride is a combined serotonin and norepinephrine (noradrenaline) reuptake inhibitor which is used to treat stress incontinence in women. Duloxetine is thought to work by increasing the tone of the urethral sphincter during filling/storage via its action on serotonin and norepinephrine in the spinal cord. Duloxetine can be used to treat moderate-to-severe stress incontinence, and has been shown to reduce the frequency of episodes of leakage. It may be more effective if combined with pelvic floor exercises. Duloxetine is approved for use in Europe, but not in the USA.

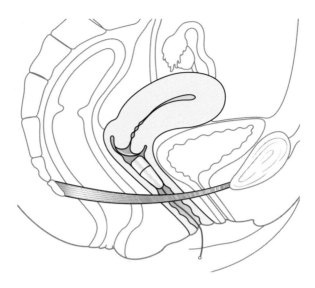

Figure 3.2 Vaginal cones are designed to help women develop awareness of the pelvic floor musculature and to strengthen the muscles. Starting with the lightest cone, the woman has to contract the pelvic floor muscles to keep the cone in position.

Surgery for stress incontinence in women should be considered only after the cause of the incontinence has been definitely ascertained. Women need to be adequately counseled about the risks and benefits of surgery for stress incontinence so that they can make an informed decision before embarking on this sort of surgery.

Surgery for stress incontinence has changed over the last 10 years with the advent of minimally invasive techniques. The gold-standard procedure for treating stress incontinence used to be colposuspension (described below), which is major surgery that necessitates a lengthy hospital stay and has a prolonged recovery time.

Sling insertion and colposuspension are not appropriate for women who may want to have more children.

Minimally invasive mid-urethral sling insertion is becoming increasingly popular, as the procedure can usually be carried out on a day-case basis, complication rates are low and long-term results are excellent (up to 85% cure rate at up to 10 years). A number of different types of sling are available and are associated with varying degrees of success.

The principle underlying the procedure is that stress incontinence is caused by failure of the pubourethral ligaments. The sling provides support under the urethra without lifting it from its anatomic position. Tension-free vaginal tape (TVT) has been most fully evaluated, and long-term follow-up data are available. The tape is made from a monofilament polypropylene knitted mesh with a large pore size. The TVT procedure was first described in 1996 and has been widely adopted for the treatment of stress incontinence. In the original technique, the sling was placed under the mid-urethra and the ends tunneled through the retropubic space (Figure 3.3) without fixation, the tape being held in position by the tissues until it becomes incorporated. However, major complications such as bowel and vascular injuries were reported, and perforation of the bladder was not uncommon (it could be managed by repositioning of the needles and postoperative bladder drainage). Other complications included erosion of the mesh through the vagina and urethra.

The transobturator mid-urethral sling (Figure 3.3) was introduced to overcome some of the problems described above. The sling is placed in a similar way to the TVT but the ends of the tape are tunneled through the obturator foramen instead of going through the retropubic space. The main advantage of this technique is that the abdominal cavity is never entered, therefore decreasing the risk of bowel injury. There are few long-term follow-up data on this method as yet, and it is not known whether the reduction in the rate of bowel injury may be negated by reduced success rates and postoperative nerve pain.

Other types of sling are also available. It is worth noting that complication rates are higher with tapes made from materials other than polypropylene. For this reason, the UK's National Institute for Health and Clinical Excellence (NICE) has recently recommended that all slings for the treatment of stress incontinence should be composed of type 1 polypropylene mesh (knitted meshes with a large pore size).

Colposuspension provides long-term cure in 70–80% of women at 10 years. It involves elevating the bladder neck by placing sutures between the lateral vaginal fornices and the ileopectineal ligament on the back of the pubic symphysis, and can be performed via an abdominal incision or laparoscopically. One of the benefits of

(a)

(b)

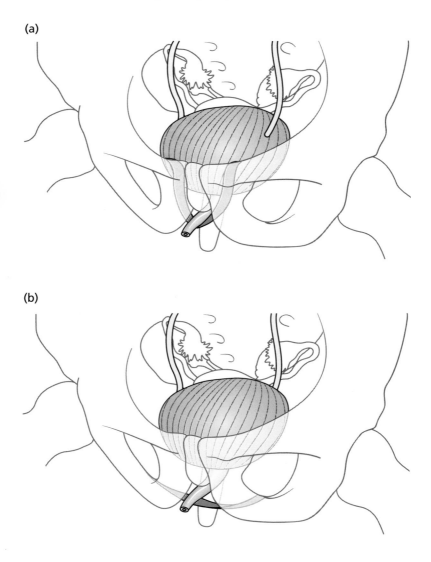

Figure 3.3 Positions of (a) retropubic and (b) transobturator mid-urethral slings to provide support for the urethra.

colposuspension is that it elevates the anterior vaginal wall and is therefore appropriate when incontinence is associated with cystocele. However, it is a more invasive procedure than sling insertion, and is associated with enterocele formation and higher rates of voiding dysfunction in the postoperative period.

Injection of bulking agents (Figure 3.4) into the urethra aids continence by opposing the walls of the urethra. Agents that can be used include collagen and silicone particles suspended in a viscous gel (Macroplastique). In the past, phenol, Teflon and fat have been used, but with poor results. A number of new materials have recently been introduced or are under development.

Bulking agents can be injected under local anesthesia and provide a treatment for women who are unfit to undergo general anesthesia or for whom a sling insertion or colposuspension are not suitable. Success

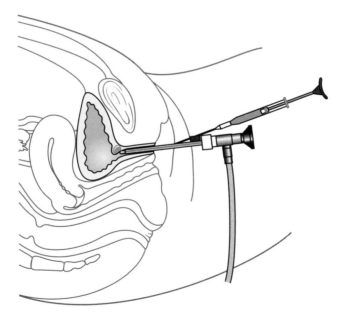

Figure 3.4 Injection of bulking agent. The agent is injected just beneath the mucosa of the urethra at the level of the bladder neck and proximal urethra, closing the bladder neck and restoring urinary continence.

rates are around 25–50% (lower than with mid-urethral slings and colposuspension), and the procedure may need to be repeated.

Other procedures. Historically a number of other operations have been used to treat stress incontinence in women. These include:

- anterior repair
- fascial slings
- Stamey procedure
- Marshall–Marchetti–Krantz procedure.

These procedures are rarely performed nowadays because the success rates and complications are worse than with minimally invasive sling insertion and colposuspension.

Complications. All surgical procedures for stress incontinence carry the risk of voiding problems in the immediate postoperative period. Patients may be unable to pass urine or completely empty their bladders for days or weeks after surgery. A number of different methods of management are available should this occur. A temporary indwelling urethral or suprapubic catheter can be placed until the bladder recovers, or the patient can be taught intermittent self-catheterization (see Chapter 9, pages 90–1). If the patient experiences voiding difficulty after TVT insertion, it is possible to loosen the tape in the early postoperative period (within 10 days), which usually resolves the problem.

Detrusor overactivity may be precipitated or worsened as a result of surgery for stress incontinence, particularly in women with bladder outlet obstruction. It is therefore important that women with mixed symptoms receive adequate counseling before consenting to surgery.

Management of stress/sphincteric incontinence in men

Stress incontinence after radical prostatectomy usually improves spontaneously. Initial management involves strengthening the pelvic floor musculature with pelvic floor exercises (see Box 3.1, page 37). Most patients improve over a period of weeks or months without the need for further investigation or treatment. Any patient who is still experiencing intractable incontinence 6 months after prostatectomy should have their sphincter function investigated urodynamically. If a clinical and urodynamic diagnosis of sphincter weakness is confirmed

Key points – urinary incontinence

- Stress incontinence is the involuntary leakage of urine on exertion. It is far more common in women than in men.
- Risk factors for stress incontinence in women include pregnancy, childbirth, menopause and obesity. Prostatectomy is the main cause in men.
- Behavioral modification, including pelvic floor exercises, is effective in women when taught correctly, and a number of devices are available to assist with training.
- The surgical procedure of choice in women is insertion of a retropubic or transobturator tape mid-urethral sling to provide support for the urethra.
- Other alternatives in women are colposuspension and injection of bulking agents.
- Options for management in men include injection of bulking agent into the urethral sphincter and insertion of a perineal sling or artificial sphincter.

and the bladder storage capacity is adequate at low pressure, the treatment options are:
- injection of bulking agents into the sphincter
- perineal sling
- insertion of an artificial sphincter.

Injectable bulking agents can be used to treat male stress incontinence. Injection suburothelially just distal to the bladder neck by cystoscopy may close the urethra sufficiently to provide continence without affecting voiding, although results vary from clinician to clinician.

Perineal sling. This minimally invasive procedure involves placing a compressive sling at the level of the bulbar urethra. The sling is anchored to the descending pubic rami, most commonly with bone screws. Success rates following radical prostatectomy range from 39% to 80%, with few complications.

Artificial urinary sphincter. Insertion of an artificial urinary sphincter (Figure 3.5) is a definitive treatment for intractable stress incontinence after prostatectomy, provided that the bladder pressure during filling is normal and that the patient is sufficiently fit to undergo surgery and is able to operate the artificial sphincter. The sphincter should be fitted at least 1 year after prostatectomy. It is activated about 6 weeks after insertion, allowing time for the tissue around the cuff to settle and for the natural capsule around each of the components to form. When the sphincter is activated, the patient has to learn to use the sphincter by compressing the pump that causes the cuff to empty. It will then automatically refill from the reservoir over a period of 1–3 minutes.

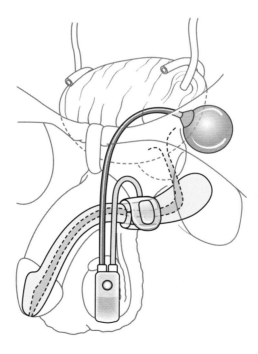

Figure 3.5 The artificial urinary sphincter. The sphincter cuff fits around the bladder neck or urethra and fills with fluid when activated, thereby passively compressing the urethra. To allow voiding, the pump is squeezed two or three times to open the cuff and transfer the fluid to the reservoir. The cuff automatically refills within 1–3 minutes.

The most common complications with artificial sphincters are infection, erosion and mechanical problems, although these problems are becoming less common as the materials and devices improve.

Key references

Bezerra CA, Bruschini H, Cody DJ. Traditional suburethral sling operations for urinary incontinence in women. *Cochrane Database Syst Rev* 2005, issue 3. CD001754. www.thecochranelibrary.com

Freeman RM. Initial management of stress urinary incontinence: pelvic floor muscle training and duloxetine. *BJOG* 2006;113(Suppl 1):10–16.

Gousse AE, Madjar S, Lambert MM, Fishman IJ. Artificial urinary sphincter for post-radical prostatectomy urinary incontinence: long-term subjective results. *J Urol* 2001;166:1755–8.

Latthe PM, Foon R, Toozs-Hobson P. Transobturator and retropubic tape procedures in stress urinary incontinence: a systematic review and meta-analysis of effectiveness and complications. *BJOG* 2007;114:522–31.

National Institute for Health and Clinical Excellence. *Urinary incontinence: the management of urinary incontinence in women.* Clinical guideline 40. London: NICE, October 2006. www.nice.org.uk\cg40

Wein AJ, Moy ML. Voiding function, dysfunction and urinary incontinence. In: Hanno P, Wein AJ, Malkowicz SB, eds. *Penn Clinical Manual of Urology.* Philadelphia: Saunders/Elsevier, 2007:341–478.

4 The overactive bladder

The term 'overactive bladder' (OAB) is defined as urgency, with or without urge incontinence, usually with frequency and nocturia. The incidence of symptomatic bladder overactivity varies with age, from about 5% in those aged 18–44 years to 20% in those over 44 years of age. Although historically thought of as a condition in women, the prevalence of OAB is in fact only slightly lower in men than in women. A greater proportion of women with OAB have urge incontinence (OAB-wet) than do men, who predominantly have OAB-dry.

The term detrusor overactivity refers to a urodynamic observation of involuntary detrusor contractions during the filling phase, which may be spontaneous or provoked. It can only be diagnosed after urodynamic investigation. Not all patients with symptoms of OAB will be found to have detrusor overactivity, and not all patients with detrusor overactivity will have symptoms of bladder overactivity.

Etiology

Overactivity can be the result of neurological abnormalities in which involuntary detrusor contractions (detrusor overactivity) occur in the presence of underlying neuropathy (e.g. multiple sclerosis, spinal cord injury or spina bifida).

Bladder overactivity can also be idiopathic, occurring in a neurologically normal individual. This is by far the most common category but, as the name implies, it is not fully understood. Overactivity is seen commonly in association with bladder outlet obstruction (i.e. together with prostatic obstruction in men, or after surgery for incontinence in women).

Investigation

It is important to exclude causes such as urinary tract infection (UTI), which can be detected with a urine dipstick test, and culture if indicated.

A frequency/volume chart (see Figure 2.2, page 21) is a reliable method of quantifying urinary frequency and volume. It also gives a good indication of fluid intake. Charts must be kept for at least 3 days to allow for variations in normal activities, but the ideal duration is not known. The chart for a patient with OAB will show frequent, irregular, small-volume voids.

Urodynamic studies are rarely indicated initially in patients who have symptoms suggestive of OAB, and most patients receive empirical treatment whether or not urodynamic studies show detrusor overactivity. The only real role for these tests in patients with OAB symptoms is if conservative therapy fails and more invasive treatment is contemplated.

Urodynamic investigation is necessary for the diagnosis of detrusor overactivity. The classic findings on multichannel cystometry are involuntary increases in detrusor pressure during filling. It is important to note, however, that only approximately 50% of patients with symptoms of detrusor overactivity will have an abnormality on supine slow-filling cystometry. Additional provocative procedures during filling, such as coughing and changes in posture, may reveal detrusor overactivity. If symptoms suggest detrusor overactivity but filling cystometry reveals a stable bladder, ambulatory urodynamic studies over a period of 4–6 hours can often reveal the detrusor dysfunction. A typical cystometry trace from a patient with detrusor overactivity is shown in Figure 2.4, page 27.

Management

The management of OAB is summarized in Table 4.1.

Lifestyle changes

Alteration in fluid intake. There is a common misconception that a fluid intake of up to 3 liters/day is needed for good health, and this becomes apparent in the frequency/volume charts of many patients. Reduction in fluid intake can bring about a dramatic improvement in patients with OAB. The ideal fluid intake for an adult is 2–2.5 liters/day.

Reduction in caffeine intake. A trial of caffeine-intake reduction is indicated in all patients presenting with OAB symptoms. It is worth noting that caffeine is present in tea, cola and chocolate, as well as coffee.

TABLE 4.1

Management of overactive bladder

- Lifestyle changes
  - Modify fluid intake to 2–2.5 liters/day
  - Reduce caffeine intake
  - Weight loss
- Behavioral therapy – bladder training
- Acupuncture (useful in some patients)
- Pharmacological therapy
  - Antimuscarinic drugs (see Table 4.3)
  - Injection of botulinum toxin into the detrusor muscle (see Figure 4.1)
- Neuromodulation
- Sacral nerve stimulation (see Figure 4.2)
- Surgery
  - Augmentation cystoplasty (rarely performed nowadays)
  - Detrusor myomectomy

Weight loss. There is evidence to suggest that weight loss can help with the symptoms of OAB in overweight patients. It is therefore worth advising weight loss to any patient who has a body mass index above 30 kg/m^2.

Behavioral therapy helps an individual to learn new patterns of response to fit in with what is considered normal. Women with OAB symptoms usually void more frequently than normal because of urgency, or to avoid situations where urgency is likely to cause a problem. In bladder training, the individual actively attempts to increase the interval between the first desire to void and the actual void. Bladder training techniques may involve mandatory schemes, where the patient is not allowed to use the toilet between set times for voiding, or self-regulated schemes, where patients attempt to increase the time interval between voids but may use the toilet in between if the urge becomes unbearable. Bladder training has been shown to be beneficial, and a course lasting for a minimum of 6 weeks, together with pelvic floor physiotherapy and exercises (see Box 3.1, page 37), should be offered as first-line treatment.

Complementary therapies include treatments that are not part of the traditional biomedical model, such as acupuncture, relaxation, meditation and herbal remedies. Acupuncture has been reported to reduce symptoms in both men and women with OAB, but there is a lack of controlled studies and skilled practitioners.

Pharmacological therapy

Antimuscarinic drugs are the mainstay of treatment for symptoms of OAB and detrusor overactivity. These drugs are classically thought to act by blocking the muscarinic receptors on the detrusor muscle that are stimulated by acetylcholine released by activated parasympathetic nerves, thereby reducing the ability of the bladder to contract. It should be noted, however, that these drugs work mainly during the storage phase, decreasing urgency and increasing bladder capacity, when there is normally no parasympathetic input into the lower urinary tract.

The effects of antimuscarinic drugs in patients with OAB symptoms are shown in Table 4.2. Treatment should be for 2–4 weeks in the first instance and can be continued if there is benefit and the side effects are tolerable; however, there is lack of evidence for how long treatment should be continued. It appears to be good practice to try discontinuing

TABLE 4.2

Effects of antimuscarinic drugs in patients with overactive bladder symptoms

- Decrease in episodes of urgency and urge incontinence
- Increase in bladder volume before the first involuntary bladder contraction
- Decrease in strength of involuntary detrusor contractions
- Increase in total bladder capacity

the drug after some months to see if bladder retraining has occurred and symptoms are improved.

Side effects of antimuscarinic drugs include dry mouth, blurred vision, changes in mental state (restlessness, disorientation, hallucinations, convulsions), nausea and constipation. Antimuscarinics are contraindicated in patients with closed-angle glaucoma or myasthenia gravis.

Oxybutynin is the most commonly used antimuscarinic. It acts both as a muscarinic antagonist and as a smooth muscle relaxant. Initially it was available as an immediate-release preparation, at a dose of 2.5–5 mg three times daily. Newer extended-release oxybutynin delivers the drug at a constant rate over a 24-hour period and can be given in doses of 5–30 mg daily. It has a better side-effect profile than the immediate-release formulation.

Transdermal administration of oxybutynin avoids first-pass liver metabolism and improves tolerability. Patches deliver a dose of 3.9 mg daily and are replaced twice weekly.

Second-generation antimuscarinics (Table 4.3) were developed to reduce the side effects experienced with oxybutynin whilst maintaining its clinical effectiveness. These drugs are more expensive than oxybutynin but they cause fewer side effects, and some require only once-daily administration, which helps with compliance.

Treatment with a second-generation antimuscarinic should ideally last for at least 1 month. Efficacy seems roughly similar between products, producing 60–75% reduction in urge incontinence episodes. If no benefit is seen, urodynamic studies should be performed before contemplating more invasive treatments.

Botulinum toxin (BTX) has the potential to revolutionize the management of refractory detrusor overactivity. It is injected directly into the detrusor muscle or suburothelially via a cystoscope (Figure 4.1), under local or general anesthesia, and acts by inhibiting neurotransmitter release, which decreases muscle contractility. There are two subtypes of BTX: BTX-A and BTX-B; the former is more widely used. BTX has been shown to be effective in the treatment of detrusor overactivity within 1–2 weeks of administration. The effect is reversible, and regeneration takes place over a period of 5–9 months, which means

TABLE 4.3

Antimuscarinic agents used in the treatment of overactive bladder

Drug	Chemical structure and primary action	Usual dosage
Darifenacin	• Tertiary amine • Relatively selective M_3 antagonist	• 7.5 or 15 mg once daily
Oxybutynin	• Tertiary amine • Relatively selective M_1/M_3 antagonist • Some calcium antagonist properties	• Immediate release: 2.5 or 5 mg twice or three times daily • Sustained release: 5–30 mg once daily
Propiverine*	• Tertiary amine • Balanced muscarinic receptor antagonist • Some calcium antagonist properties	• 15 mg twice or three times daily
Solifenacin	• Tertiary amine • Relatively selective M_3/M_1 antagonist	• 5 or 10 mg once daily
Tolterodine	• Tertiary amine • Balanced muscarinic receptor antagonist	• Immediate-release: 1 or 2 mg twice daily • Sustained release: 2 or 4 mg once daily
Trospium	• Quaternary amine • Balanced muscarinic receptor antagonist	• 20 mg twice daily[†]

*Not available in the USA.
[†]Once-daily formulation (60 g dose) is being developed.

that repeated injections may be necessary. The most important potential adverse effects are detrusor hypotonia and urinary retention. Although widely used, BTX does not yet have regulatory approval for this indication in the USA or the UK, but trials are in progress. The exact dosage, number of injections per treatment and sites of injection for neurogenic and idiopathic OAB have yet to be standardized.

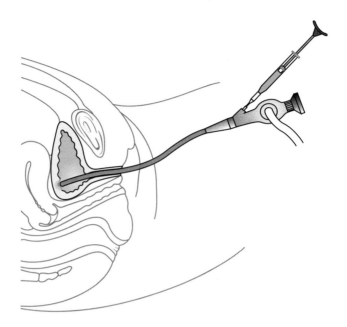

Figure 4.1 Botulinum toxin is injected via a cystoscope directly into the detrusor muscle.

Neuromodulation involves the electrical stimulation of a peripheral nerve or the spinal cord and is thought to improve the ability to suppress detrusor contractions. It is being used increasingly in the treatment of refractory detrusor overactivity. The various techniques for neuromodulation include removable peripheral nerve stimulators and implantable sacral nerve stimulators. Overall, electrical neurostimulation and neuromodulation have a 30–50% clinical success rate.

Sacral nerve stimulation (Figure 4.2) differs from other forms of neuromodulation in that it provides continuous stimulation via an implanted pulse generator connected to an electrode within the S3 foramina. Its mode of action is not entirely clear, but results in this difficult-to-treat group of patients appear promising. Sacral nerve stimulation has been shown to be safe, effective and durable.

Transvaginal electrical stimulation has been shown to be better than placebo.

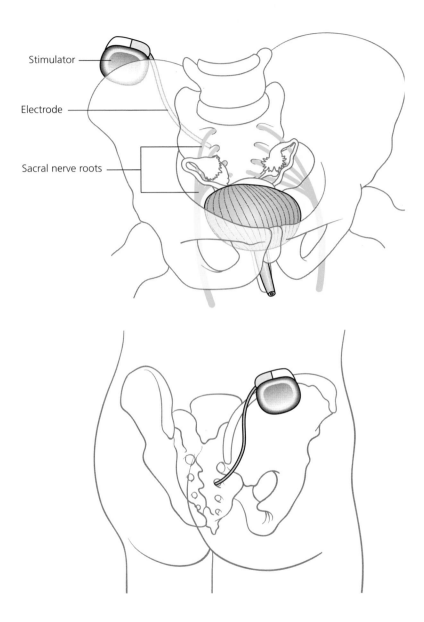

Stimulator

Electrode

Sacral nerve roots

Figure 4.2 Sacral nerve stimulation provides continuous stimulation via an implanted pulse generator connected to an electrode within the S3 foramina.

53

Key points – the overactive bladder

- Overactive bladder (OAB) describes a condition in which the patient experiences urgency, with or without urge incontinence, usually with frequency and nocturia.
- Detrusor overactivity refers to involuntary detrusor contractions during filling; diagnosis is by urodynamic investigation.
- Bladder overactivity can be neurogenic or idiopathic. Idiopathic OAB can be associated with bladder outlet obstruction.
- A frequency/volume chart is useful in diagnosis.
- Initial management includes behavioral modification.
- Antimuscarinic drugs are a mainstay of conservative treatment.
- Surgical options include augmentation cystoplasty and the newer technique of detrusor myomectomy.

Surgery

Augmentation cystoplasty used to be the gold standard in the surgical treatment of detrusor overactivity but is now rarely necessary, except in cases of neuropathic overactivity that is refractory to all other treatment modalities. The procedure involves opening the bladder and stitching in a piece of compliant tissue, usually a loop of detubularized ileum on a vascular pedicle, to increase the bladder capacity and compliance. The bladder remains overactive, but when it contracts the improved compliance means that lower intravesical pressures are generated, protecting the upper tracts from the effects of high intravesical pressure. Urge incontinence is also reduced.

Because the bladder contractility is reduced, there is a high risk of postoperative urinary retention, and patients should be counseled about the possibility of self-catheterization before undergoing surgery (see pages 90–1).

When bowel has been used to augment the bladder, the mucosa continues to secrete mucus, which is passed with the urine and can lead to retention. There is also a risk of stone formation and malignant change in the transposed segment of bowel.

This procedure is most commonly used when the upper urinary tract is at risk from damage due to increased intravesical pressure, which is most common in the neuropathic bladder (see Chapter 9).

Detrusor myomectomy has recently been suggested as an alternative to augmentation cystoplasty. It involves removal of the detrusor muscle from the dome of the bladder, leaving the mucosa intact, in effect creating a large bladder diverticulum. This allows bladder capacity to increase and lowers the intravesical pressure. This technique circumvents the potential complications of mucus retention, stone formation and malignant change seen with cystoplasty. However, it is a relatively new procedure and the long-term results are not yet known.

Key references

Alhasso A, Glazener CMA, Pickard R, N'Dow J. Adrenergic drugs for urinary incontinence in adults. *Cochrane Database Syst Rev* 2005, issue 3. CD001842. www.thecochranelibrary.com

MacDiarmid S, Rogers A. Male overactive bladder: the role of urodynamics and anticholinergics. *Curr Urol Rep* 2007;8:66–73.

Schurch B. Botulinum toxin for the management of bladder dysfunction. *Drugs* 2006;66:1301–18.

Voiding problems occur when there is an impediment to the normal smooth emptying of the bladder. This may result from obstruction to the normal bladder outflow – the focus of this chapter – alone or in combination with impaired contractility of the detrusor muscle.

Bladder outlet obstruction

Outlet obstruction may occur at any point along the length of the urethra from the bladder neck to the urethral meatus. The likely causes are listed in Table 5.1. The most common cause is benign prostatic enlargement secondary to hyperplasia. The patient may present with a variety of storage and voiding symptoms.

Etiology and risk factors

Benign prostatic hyperplasia (BPH) refers to a regional nodular growth of varying combinations of glandular and stromal proliferation that occurs in almost all men who have testes and who live long enough. The term encompasses histological cellular proliferation (microscopic BPH) and consequent prostate enlargement (macroscopic BPH). The term BPE indicates benign prostatic enlargement, usually due to BPH, while BPO indicates benign prostatic obstruction, a common cause of bladder outlet obstruction.

Microscopic BPH is seen in about 25% of men aged 40–50 years, 50% of men aged 50–60 years, 65% of men aged 60–70 years, 80% of men aged 70–80 years and 90% of men aged 80–90 years. It is estimated that 25–50% of men with microscopic and macroscopic BPH (BPE) will develop filling/storage symptoms, alone or in combination with voiding symptoms, mainly due to BPO. However, far fewer men complain about these symptoms than of BPH, and even fewer seek help because of these symptoms.

The cause of BPH is not fully understood. The hormonal theory postulates that estrogen–androgen synergism associated with aging drives prostatic growth.

TABLE 5.1

Causes of bladder outlet obstruction

Congenital

- Posterior urethral valves
- Urethral stricture
- Ectopic ureterocele

Acquired

- Structural
  - Benign prostatic enlargement
  - Prostatic carcinoma
  - Bladder neck obstruction
  - Urethral stricture
  - Urethral stones
  - External compression
  - Pelvic floor prolapse
- Functional
  - Detrusor–sphincter dyssynergia
  - Detrusor atony (contributing factor)

Posterior urethral valves are a congenital cause of bladder outlet obstruction in boys, which, if severe, can lead to hydronephrosis and renal failure. One in every 5000–8000 boys is born with posterior urethral valves.

Urethral stricture is an abnormal narrowing of the urethra that causes obstruction to the outflow of urine and may ultimately lead to back pressure on the bladder, ureters and kidneys. Strictures may be caused by inflammation or scarring as a result of surgery, disease or injury. The risk is increased in patients with sexually transmitted diseases, repeated episodes of urethritis or BPH. Instrumentation of the urethra (with a catheter or cystoscope) also increases the risk. Congenital strictures and true strictures occur rarely in women.

Primary bladder neck obstruction is thought to occur as a result of congenital constriction, or failure to open that is not associated with the urethra. It is characterized by incomplete opening of the bladder neck during voluntary or involuntary voiding. It is found almost exclusively in young and middle-aged men, and is characterized by long-standing storage and voiding symptoms. These men typically have normal-sized prostate glands, and objective evidence of obstruction is easily obtained on urodynamic examination. Once obstruction is diagnosed, it may be located to the bladder neck by videourodynamic investigation or urethral-pressure profiling. The diagnosis may also be made on the grounds of outlet obstruction in the absence of urethral stricture, prostatic enlargement or detrusor–sphincter dyssynergia (DSD).

Secondary bladder neck obstruction may be caused by posterior urethral valves and results from hypertrophy of the bladder neck muscle in response to increased voiding pressure caused by the urethral abnormality.

Symptoms of bladder outlet obstruction vary. The most common symptoms are listed in Table 5.2.

Examination and investigations. A thorough abdominal and pelvic examination should be carried out to evaluate the following:
- bladder distension
- abdominal mass
- prostatic enlargement and presence/absence of nodularity or induration (digital rectal examination [Figure 5.1] is mandatory in men and has been shown to be an accurate predictor of prostate size)
- prolapse, particularly cystocele, in women.

TABLE 5.2

Common symptoms suggestive of bladder outlet obstruction

- Slow urinary flow
- Delayed onset of urination (urinary hesitancy)
- Inability to urinate (acute urinary retention)
- Urine stream that starts and stops (urinary intermittency)
- Urgency/frequency
- Urge incontinence
- Nocturia
- Continuous feeling of a full bladder

In addition, urinalysis should be performed to detect hematuria (see Chapter 6) and signs of infection, and serum creatinine should be measured. Some men with BPH will have some degree of renal impairment. It is important to investigate this, as it affects clinical management. For example, a man with BPH and renal impairment may require more urgent surgical intervention and will need to be monitored more closely during and after surgery.

There is some debate about whether the measurement of prostate-specific antigen (PSA) is mandatory. This issue is beyond the scope of this book; however, it would seem sensible to measure the serum PSA in all men with a life expectancy of more than 5 years and in whom the diagnosis of prostate cancer would influence treatment decisions. Ideally, the advantages and disadvantages of such testing should be explained to the patient.

Uroflowmetry and urodynamic investigation. Measurement of urinary flow rate is an extremely useful investigation in patients with voiding dysfunction. The reduced flow rate characteristic of prostatic

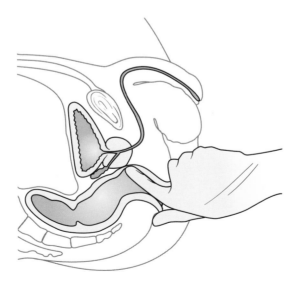

Figure 5.1 Digital rectal examination of the prostate is mandatory for men with lower urinary tract symptoms, and has been shown to be an accurate predictor of prostate size.

outlet obstruction is shown in Figure 2.3, page 25. Urodynamically, outlet obstruction is generally defined as high detrusor pressure accompanied by low urine flow rate. Once obstruction has been diagnosed, videourodynamic investigation can be useful to determine the site of the obstruction.

Urodynamic studies are not indicated for all men suspected of having BPH. They are most useful to differentiate outlet obstruction from impaired detrusor contractility, and should be performed in patients with equivocal findings in whom invasive therapy is being considered.

Transrectal ultrasonography can be helpful if an accurate size estimate is desired and when clinical findings or PSA levels suggest the presence of prostate cancer. It is also used to guide prostatic biopsy.

Measurement of postvoid residual volume may be a useful aid in the management of patients with outlet obstruction, but it may vary quite a lot in a given individual.

Management of voiding disorders

Bladder outlet obstruction secondary to benign prostatic obstruction. The aim of treatment is to relieve the obstruction by reducing the smooth muscle tone or bulk of the prostate.

Selective α-1 adrenoceptor antagonists have been shown to increase peak urinary flow rates and improve symptoms in 30–45% of men, but they are of little value in patients with complete inability to void. They act by relaxing the prostate and bladder neck smooth muscle, reducing outlet obstruction without adversely affecting detrusor contractility.

5α-reductase inhibitors block the conversion of testosterone to dihydrotestosterone, which plays a key role in the development of BPH. These drugs can potentially reverse or arrest the process of BPH and have been shown to reduce prostate volume by up to 20% over 6–10 months.

Surgical treatment of BPH has the best results in terms of improvement in symptoms and urine flow rates, but is associated with a much higher incidence of complications than medical treatment.

Transurethral resection of the prostate (Figure 5.2) is the most common surgical treatment for BPH. The prostate is resected with a diathermy loop in a resectoscope inserted via the urethra. Symptom relief is achieved in 70–90% of men. The most significant complications are erectile dysfunction in 2–5%, incontinence in 0.2–1% and retrograde ejaculation in 70–90% of men.

Transurethral incision of the bladder neck and prostate is used when a patient has obstruction caused by a prostate that is relatively small (generally less than 35 g), with a high bladder neck and no hyperplasia of the middle lobe. The procedure involves making an incision through the bladder neck from just below the level of the ureteric orifices to a point about 0.1 cm proximal to the verumontanum. It is almost as effective as transurethral resection but with lower complication rates, although the likelihood that further treatment may become necessary is higher.

Laser ablation of the prostate is an alternative to transurethral resection. It involves vaporization of the enlarged prostate with a neodynium, yttrium or holmium laser. This procedure may have advantages over the traditional transurethral resection as it causes less bleeding and the hospital stay is generally shorter, while the short-term outcomes are similar.

Open prostatectomy is indicated only in men who have extremely large prostates.

(a)   (b)

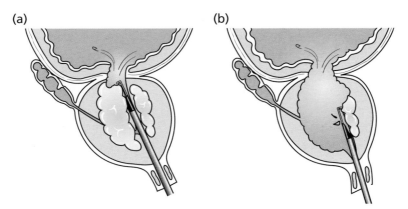

Figure 5.2 Transurethral resection of the prostate. (a) The median lobe is resected; (b) lateral adenoma tissue is removed, leaving a cavity that subsequently epithelializes over 4–6 weeks.

Primary bladder neck obstruction. Although α-1 adrenoceptor antagonists provide some relief in patients with bladder neck dysfunction, definitive relief is best achieved in men by bladder neck incision. Surgery should be carried out with caution in the rare woman with primary bladder neck obstruction, as the risk of postoperative urinary incontinence after bladder neck incision is high.

Urethral stricture. Treatment is initially by urethral dilatation or urethrotomy, although complex or recurrent cases may require urethroplasty.

Key points – voiding problems

- Voiding problems occur when normal smooth emptying of the bladder is impeded, through obstruction or impaired detrusor contractility.
- Benign prostatic enlargement secondary to benign prostatic hyperplasia (BPH), a process of normal aging in men, is the most common cause of outlet obstruction. Rarer causes include posterior urethral valves, urethral stricture and bladder neck obstruction, which may be congenital or secondary to increased voiding pressures as a result of urethral abnormality.
- Uroflowmetry and urodynamic investigations are useful in the diagnosis of outlet obstruction but are not indicated for all men thought to have BPH. Transurethral ultrasonography and measurement of postvoid residual volume may also provide useful information.
- Obstruction due to BPH can be treated with α-1 adrenoceptor antagonists and 5α-reductase inhibitors. Surgery (transurethral resection, vaporization or incision of the prostate) may be needed.
- Surgery is often required for bladder neck obstruction and urethral stricture.

Key references

Barry MJ, Roehrborn CG. Benign prostatic hyperplasia. *BMJ* 2001;323:1042–6.

Fried NM. New laser treatment approaches for benign prostatic hyperplasia. *Curr Urol Rep* 2007;8:47–52.

Kirby RS, McConnell JD. *Fast Facts: Benign Prostatic Hyperplasia*, 5th edn. Oxford: Health Press, 2005.

Madersbacher S, Marszalek M, Lackner J et al. The long-term outcome of medical therapy for BPH. *Eur Urol* 2007;51:1522–33.

McCrery RJ, Appell RA. Bladder outlet obstruction in women: iatrogenic, anatomic, and neurogenic. *Curr Urol Rep* 2006;7:363–9.

Wein AJ, Lee DI. Benign prostatic hyperplasia and related entities. In: Hanno P, Wein AJ, Malkowicz SB, eds. *Penn Clinical Manual of Urology*. Philadelphia: Saunders/ Elsevier, 2007:479–522.

Hematuria can originate from anywhere along the urinary tract and may be an indicator of underlying pathology. It can be microscopic or macroscopic (gross), but the investigation for each is similar.

Prevalence

The prevalence of hematuria on urine dipstick testing in adults is estimated by various sources to be 2–16%. Dipstick testing is sensitive but is not specific, and it is difficult to distinguish between 'physiological' amounts of blood in the urine and blood that is the result of pathology.

Etiology

Urinary tract pathology is found in 2–10% of patients under the age of 50 years with microscopic hematuria. The most common pathologies are stones, infection, nephritis and, in men, prostate enlargement (see page 56). Urinary tract malignancy is rarely seen in patients under 40 years of age. Over 50 years, 10–20% of patients with microscopic hematuria will have significant urinary tract pathology. Malignancy is more common in this age group when there is gross hematuria.

History

In taking a history it is important to distinguish hematuria from rectal bleeding, and from vaginal bleeding in women. A history of urinary frequency and dysuria would suggest an infectious cause, which is the most common cause of hematuria in young women. Urinary tract calculi may present with pain. Glomerulonephritis or nephropathy may occur secondary to a recent upper respiratory tract infection, rash or edema.

Drugs may cause hematuria: non-steroidal anti-inflammatory drugs can cause papillary necrosis, while danazol and cyclophosphamide can cause hemorrhagic cystitis. Anticoagulants will not cause hematuria unless the person is over-anticoagulated.

Bladder tumors classically present with painless frank hematuria. Risk factors for bladder tumors are shown in Table 6.1.

TABLE 6.1

Risk factors for bladder tumors

- Smoking
- Exposure to chemicals or dyes (benzenes or aromatic amines)
- Chemotherapy with cyclosphosphamide or ifosfamide
- *Shistosoma hematobium* infection
- Chronic irritation and infection
- Pelvic irradiation
- Age over 40 years

Investigations

Flow charts for the investigation of hematuria are shown in Figures 6.1 and 6.2.

Microscopy. Hematuria identified by dipstick urinalysis should always be investigated further by urine microscopy. Microscopic hematuria is present if more than three red blood cells per high-power field are visible in urinary sediment from two out of three freshly voided, clean-catch midstream urine samples. The incidence of hematuria on microscopy varies from 0.2% to 16.1% in population-based studies.

Microscopy can also provide further information about the morphology of the red blood cells. Misshapen red blood cells are usually glomerular in origin, whereas normal red blood cells generally come from the lower urinary tract. Red blood cell casts are almost always associated with glomerular disease.

Urine culture is vital to exclude infection as a cause of hematuria; hematuria should never be attributed to infection without a positive culture. In the case of urine infection, a specimen should be examined after treatment to exclude continuing hematuria.

Biochemistry. Urine should be tested for proteinuria, which may be a sign of renal pathology or an extrarenal medical disorder. If proteinuria is identified, serum urea, creatinine and electrolytes should be measured.

Urine cytology is helpful in the diagnosis of transitional cell carcinoma. It is important to note, however, that sensitivity varies from less than 20% to over 90% depending on the tumor grade, sensitivity being lowest for well-differentiated tumors.

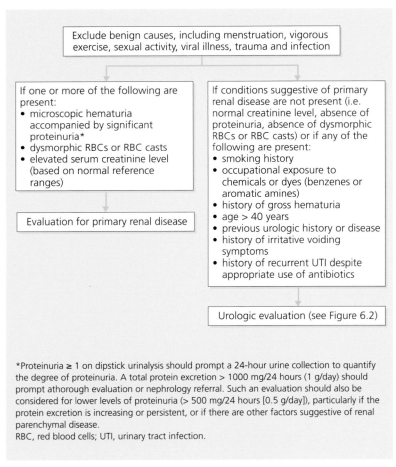

*Proteinuria ≥ 1 on dipstick urinalysis should prompt a 24-hour urine collection to quantify the degree of proteinuria. A total protein excretion > 1000 mg/24 hours (1 g/day) should prompt athorough evaluation or nephrology referral. Such an evaluation should also be considered for lower levels of proteinuria (> 500 mg/24 hours [0.5 g/day]), particularly if the protein excretion is increasing or persistent, or if there are other factors suggestive of renal parenchymal disease.
RBC, red blood cells; UTI, urinary tract infection.

Figure 6.1 Initial evaluation of patients with newly diagnosed asymptomatic microscopic hematuria. The recommended definition of microscopic hematuria is three or more red blood cells per high-power field on microscopic evaluation of two of three properly collected specimens. Adapted from American Urology Association guidelines for the assessment and treatment of asymptomatic hematuria. Grossfeld et al. 2001.

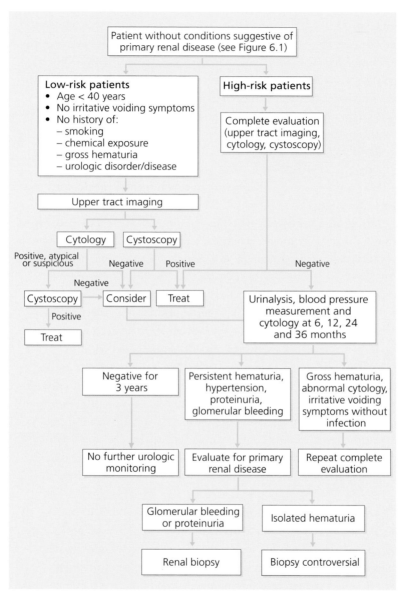

Figure 6.2 Diagnosis of hematuria in patients without conditions suggestive of primary renal disease. Adapted from American Urology Association guidelines for the assessment and treatment of asymptomatic hematuria. Grossfeld et al. 2001.

Imaging

Ultrasonography of the renal tract is the preferred initial imaging technique for identifying renal parenchymal disease, hydronephrosis and stone fragments. If hydronephrosis is found, the entire renal tract should be investigated. Ultrasonography can be used to detect and characterize renal masses but is unreliable in detecting upper tract urothelial tumors.

Plain abdominal radiography is useful to detect calcification due to renal tract stones, which affect about 5% of the population. Calcification may also be seen with infection such as tuberculosis, and nephrocalcinosis.

Intravenous urography (IVU) has traditionally been the modality of choice for imaging the urinary tract, and many still consider it to be the best imaging test for the initial evaluation of microscopic hematuria. It has limited sensitivity for the detection of small renal masses and cannot differentiate between solid and cystic masses.

Computed tomography (CT) is more sensitive for detecting small renal masses and is the investigation of choice for detecting renal tract stones – it is extremely sensitive (94–98%) compared with IVU (52–59%) and ultrasonography (19%). CT is used to detect and characterize solid renal masses as well as renal and perirenal infections and associated complications. CT is therefore the most efficient investigation in differentiating the causes of hematuria and, if used as the investigation of first choice, would reduce the time taken to diagnose the underlying etiology. The sensitivity of CT urography in detecting urothelial lesions compared with IVU is not yet established.

Cystoscopy is recommended for the investigation of hematuria in adults. It allows for accurate detection of mucosal abnormalities and can be performed reliably with a flexible cystoscope under local anesthesia. It is possible to take bladder biopsies using a flexible cystoscope, although resection requires a rigid cystoscope and general anesthesia.

'One-stop' clinics. The investigation of hematuria is often carried out in 'one-stop' clinics with facilities for cytology, ultrasonography and

Key points – hematuria

- Blood in the urine can originate from anywhere along the urinary tract and may indicate underlying pathology.
- Dipstick testing is sensitive but does not distinguish between physiological and pathological amounts of blood.
- The most common causes of hematuria are stones, infection, nephritis and prostate enlargement. Malignancy becomes more likely in patients over 50 years of age. Some drugs can cause hematuria.
- The morphology of red blood cells may distinguish between glomerular and lower urinary tract causes.
- Investigation of hematuria can be in a 'one-stop' clinic with facilities for cytology, ultrasonography and flexible cystoscopy so that diagnosis can be made in one visit.
- Ultrasonography is useful for identifying renal parenchymal disease and urinary tract obstruction. Radiography will identify stones. CT scanning is highly sensitive for detecting stones, renal masses and infections.
- Management depends on the underlying cause identified.
- Unexplained hematuria should be followed up with repeat tests at a later date.

flexible cystoscopy, the aim being to make the diagnosis in a single outpatient visit.

Management

The main principles of managing hematuria are as follows.

- Infections should be managed appropriately.
- Patients with stones or renal tumors should be referred to the appropriate urologist.
- Patients with significant proteinuria, renal insufficiency, or red blood cell casts or dysmorphic red blood cells on microscopy should be referred to a nephrologist for evaluation of renal parenchymal disease, which may necessitate a percutaneous renal biopsy.

Follow-up. Investigation finds no cause for microscopic hematuria in many patients. Such unexplained hematuria presents a management dilemma. Although most units will discharge these patients, it has been suggested that repeat urinalysis, cytology and blood pressure monitoring is required. Unexplained frank hematuria requires more extensive investigation.

Key references

Grossfeld GD, Wolf JS Jr, Litwan MS et al. Asymptomatic microscopic hematuria in adults: summary of the AUA best practice policy recommendations. *Am Fam Physician* 2001;63:1145–54.

Raghavan D, Bailey M. *Fast Facts: Bladder Cancer*, 2nd edn. Oxford: Health Press, 2006.

Rodgers MA, Hempel S, Aho T et al. Diagnostic tests used in the investigation of adult haematuria. A systematic review. *BJU Int* 2006;98:1154–60.

Rodgers M, Nixon J, Hempel S et al. Diagnostic tests and algorithms used in the investigation of haematuria: systematic reviews and economic evaluation. *Health Technol Assess* 2006;10:iii–iv, xi–259.

Asymptomatic bacteriuria

Asymptomatic bacteriuria refers to the finding of a significant number of bacteria in the urine of a patient but without any of the symptoms of urinary tract infection (UTI). The prevalence varies from 5% of premenopausal women to more than 15% in the elderly; almost 100% of patients with a permanent indwelling catheter are affected.

Because of the increasing problem of bacterial resistance to antibiotics, it is important to rationalize treatment of asymptomatic bacteriuria. The majority of patients will not benefit from antibiotic treatment, and it is thus not indicated. However, it is important to treat asymptomatic infections in a small number of patient groups, as summarized in Table 7.1.

Recurrent urinary tract infection

Recurrent UTI is defined as a UTI followed by a further infection after resolution of the initial bacteriuria. Often this reinfection is caused by repeated contamination of the urinary tract with perineal flora.

Epidemiology. Women are much more susceptible to UTIs than are men; at least 20–30% of women will have a UTI at some time in their life, 25% of whom will develop recurrent UTI.

TABLE 7.1

Patient groups in whom treatment of asymptomatic bacteriuria is warranted

- Pregnant women – up to 40% will develop a kidney infection if asymptomatic bacteriuria is left untreated
- Kidney transplant recipients
- Young children with vesicoureteral reflux
- Patients with infected kidney stones

Bacteria most commonly associated with UTI are *Escherichia coli* (80%) and *Klebsiella* (5%), *Enterobacter* (2%) and *Proteus* (2%) species. *Staphylococcus saprophyticus* causes 10% of cases of acute cystitis in young women. Anaerobic infections of the urinary tract are rare.

Etiology. Table 7.2 lists underlying pathologies that should be considered, although it is unlikely that an underlying abnormality will be identified.

The normal vaginal flora inhibits the growth of *E. coli* and other Gram-negative fecal flora, possibly through the production of hydrogen peroxide. Alteration of this flora may promote the growth of bacteria that are pathogenic to the urinary tract. Glycogen stores in genital tract epithelial cells are depleted after the menopause, and the environment is less supportive of *Lactobacilli* growth. There is therefore increased colonization of the vagina with *Enterobacter* species. Vaginal pH increases after the menopause, making these women more prone to UTI.

Symptoms of lower UTI include frequency of micturition, urgency, dysuria and suprapubic discomfort. Women with lower UTI are usually systemically well, but symptoms such as fever, with or without rigors, malaise, nausea and vomiting may occur if the infection ascends. Renal angle pain and tenderness are often predominant features of pyelonephritis.

TABLE 7.2

Pathologies that may lead to recurrent urinary tract infection

- Bladder or urethral diverticulum
- Urinary tract calculi
- Bowel fistula (normally secondary to Crohn's disease, diverticulitis or radiation treatment)
- Urethral strictures/any cause of obstruction
- Carcinoma
- Incomplete bladder emptying

Diagnosis. Urinalysis using dipstick tests for leukocytes and bacterial nitrite production is quick and easy. A positive dipstick test result has sensitivity in the region of 70% and a specificity of 80% for finding significant pathogens in urine. Microscopy remains the gold standard for the diagnosis of UTI, and urine must be cultured in the presence of antimicrobials to determine sensitivities.

Investigation. The extent to which recurrent UTI should be investigated is controversial; it does, however, make sense to rule out the common pathological abnormalities. It is important to note that UTIs are relatively rare in men and are therefore more likely to have a significant cause than in women.

Tests performed can include an estimation of postvoid residual urine volume, outpatient cystoscopy and imaging of the upper urinary tract, usually with ultrasonography and plain radiography, looking for calculi, evidence of reflux and cortical scarring. However, such investigations will prove negative in the majority of patients, and a degree of clinical discretion is required to prevent the expense and distress caused by overinvestigation, particularly in young women in whom concurrent pathology is unlikely.

Further investigation will depend on clinical factors such as the coexistence of hematuria (see Chapter 6), the severity of symptoms and the presence of atypical organisms such as *P. mirabilis*, which is commonly found in association with stones.

Treatment. Any underlying cause should be treated. Patients who are found to have incomplete bladder emptying, with postvoid residual volumes that are consistently greater than 100 mL, should be taught to double void. Intermittent self-catheterization (see Chapter 9, pages 90–1) to empty the bladder fully at least once a day should be recommended for patients with large postvoid residual volumes.

Urethral dilatation has been a common treatment but there is little evidence to support its use unless a urethral stricture is present.

In rare cases of vesicoureteric reflux, submucosal injection of collagen in the ureterovesical junction or ureteric reimplantation may be indicated to protect the kidneys from damage.

The majority of investigations, however, will be normal, and treatment should be on the basis of symptoms.

Adequate fluid intake (at least 2 liters/day) will help to maintain a good urine output to flush pathogens away. Patients should void frequently and completely, and women should be advised to void before bed and after sexual intercourse.

Cranberry juice contains substances such as fructose that inhibit the adherence of some bacteria to uroepithelial cells. One report showed that drinking 300 mL cranberry juice daily reduced the incidence of bacteriuria with pyuria by 42%. Cranberry juice is acidic, so it is usually combined with water and sweeteners; the cranberry content of commercial cranberry juice drinks therefore varies somewhat. Cranberry extract tablets have also been found useful in the prophylaxis of UTIs.

Antibiotic treatment is recommended for patients with recurrent UTIs. Acute infections should be treated with a short course of an appropriate antibiotic, the type depending on local resistance. The majority of uncomplicated lower UTIs respond to a 3-day course of trimethoprim or a 7-day course of amoxicillin or nitrofurantoin. However, urine culture before treatment is important, given the widespread resistance to antibiotics. Alternative antibiotics for resistant organisms include co-amoxiclav, oral cephalosporins or a quinolone.

Antibiotic prophylaxis. A continuous regimen of low-dose antibiotics can be used as prophylaxis against further infections in selected patients. At low doses, an adequate concentration of antibiotic will be achieved in the urine but with little effect on the fecal and vaginal flora, thereby preventing the development of resistant strains and complications related to the reduction of normal flora, such as genital *Candida* infections. A single antibiotic can be used: trimethoprim, cefalexin and nitrofurantoin are commonly recommended. These remain effective in the long term despite continued use. Significant resistance does not develop, and adverse effects are rare. Some clinicians recommend a 3-monthly rotating regimen of different antimicrobials to minimize any small chance of promoting resistant strains.

Prophylactic antibiotic use reduces the frequency of infections by 95%, to a mean of fewer than 0.2 infections per year. Breakthrough infections should be treated with full doses of appropriate antibiotics.

Consideration should be given to stopping the prophylactic regimen after 6–12 months to see if the frequency of infections has altered. However, some patients may need to continue daily prophylaxis for life. An alternative to prophylaxis is to allow patients to self-medicate. Patients are provided with 3 days' full-dose antibiotic treatment to take when they experience the symptoms of acute cystitis; the symptoms of UTIs can be accurately identified by 85% of women. Postcoital antibiotics will be beneficial for some women if sexual intercourse appears to be the sole predisposing factor.

Vaginal estrogen. There is some evidence that vaginal estrogen is beneficial in postmenopausal women with recurrent UTIs. It increases the cellular glycogen concentration and encourages recolonization with *Lactobacilli*, thus reducing the vaginal pH and therefore the concentration of pathogenic bacteria.

Painful bladder syndrome and interstitial cystitis

Painful bladder syndrome (PBS) has been described by the International Continence Society as a condition in which a patient experiences suprapubic pain related to bladder filling, accompanied by other symptoms such as increased daytime and night-time frequency, in the absence of proven UTI or other obvious pathology. The diagnosis of interstitial cystitis (IC) is confined to patients with painful bladder symptoms who have characteristic cystoscopic and histological features.

Epidemiology. There is no real agreement as to the true incidence of PBS or IC, as there are no formalized diagnostic criteria. Estimates of the incidence of the latter vary from 8 to 865 per 100 000.

It is commonly accepted that IC predominates in women. Estimates of population prevalence indicate male-to-female ratios of 1:4.5 to 1:9, although few studies have included enough men to show whether there are true sex differences.

Etiology. Despite extensive scientific effort, the precise etiology of PBS and IC has yet to be explained. The initial descriptions of IC by Guy Hunner in 1918 included loss of epithelium, with the underlying

75

mucosa showing granulation tissue, increased capillaries, edema and chronic inflammatory cells, also involving the muscle coat and thickened peritoneum over the diseased area. Precisely what causes these changes is not known, and no causal agent has been found. These changes are generally considered to be late changes, and many patients with PBS/IC have no specific cystoscopic findings.

Symptoms. The diagnosis of PBS/IC is based clinically on symptoms of urinary frequency, urgency and pain. Pain is an essential component of both conditions and is traditionally described as increasing pain on bladder filling that is relieved by voiding. It is recognized that pain may present as bladder, urethral, vaginal, rectal or pelvic pain, and it may be suprapubic, urethral, perineal or a combination. There are no criteria for the nature or location of the pain except that it must be chronic and have no other obvious cause.

Diagnosis of PBS or IC requires the exclusion of other causes of the bladder symptoms, such as infection, malignancy, radiation or drug-induced cystitis.

Cystoscopy and biopsy. The 'classic' cystoscopic picture of IC is one of punctate petechial hemorrhages observed on second-look cystoscopy after cystodistension to 70–80 cmH$_2$O for 1–3 minutes. This needs to be carried out under general anesthesia; outpatient flexible cystoscopy is inadequate to make this diagnosis. These cystoscopic findings are not necessarily diagnostic, however, as not all patients with petechial hemorrhages have IC, and vice versa.

Bladder biopsy may show changes such as infiltration with inflammatory cells in all or specific parts of the bladder wall.

There is some disagreement about the role of cystoscopy and bladder biopsy in the diagnosis of IC. Some clinicians will diagnose IC in a patient who has a 3-month history of urinary urgency and frequency and a negative urinary culture and cytology, whereas others will diagnose the condition only if there are the characteristic cystoscopic findings, preferably with histological confirmation. Biopsy is only really clinically indicated if there is a suspicion of malignancy or as part of a clinical protocol.

Management. Once the diagnosis of PBS/IC is made, the next decision is whether to initiate treatment or to consider a course of 'watchful waiting'. The natural history of the disorder is not fully understood, and the proportion of patients whose symptoms will resolve spontaneously is not known. Treatment is not always necessary if a patient's symptoms are tolerable and do not impact significantly on quality of life; there are few data to show that treatment will significantly alter the natural history of the disorder.

Education and empowerment have important roles, and patients are reassured to know that their symptoms are part of a recognized syndrome that affects many people. Options for treatment are summarized in Table 7.3.

Dietary advice. Many patients find that PBS seems to be affected by particular foods, mostly 'acidic' drinks, spicy foods, caffeine and

TABLE 7.3

Treatment options* for painful bladder syndrome / interstitial cystitis

- Dietary training: identification and avoidance of dietary 'triggers' (e.g. acidic drinks, spicy foods, caffeine, alcohol)
- Bladder training
- Pharmacological treatment
  - Tricyclic antidepressants (see Table 7.4)
  - Analgesics
  - Hydroxyzine
  - Sodium pentosanpolysulfate
  - Intravesical injection of chlorpactin, dimethyl sulfoxide, heparin, hyaluronic acid, sodium pentosanpolysulfate
- Invasive treatment (if all else fails and symptoms are debilitating)
  - Sacral nerve stimulation (see Chapter 4, pages 52–3)
  - Augmentation cystoplasty (rarely)

*If management is chosen over watchful waiting.

alcohol. A wide variety of foods has been implicated and special diets for patients with IC are provided in patient information. Not all foods affect all patients in the same way so it is important to advise patients to avoid only those foods that affect them.

Behavioral changes. Bladder training may have a modest benefit in some patients with painful bladder symptoms and can reduce the frequency of voiding.

Oral treatments. The effects of therapy are difficult to evaluate, given the uncertain natural history of the condition and the fact that the condition tends to vary in severity. The following drugs have been reported to be beneficial.

Tricyclic antidepressants used in the treatment of IC are listed in Table 7.4. Amitriptyline is commonly used for its analgesic properties, although the mechanism of action is not known. It has been used in the treatment of IC and is useful in the management of pain at a dose of 75 mg daily. Its effectiveness is limited by side effects of drowsiness, fatigue, weight gain and dry mouth – approximately one-third of patients cannot tolerate amitriptyline.

Analgesics. The appropriate long-term use of analgesics plays an integral role in the conservative management of PBS. Most patients can be helped by using medications used for chronic neuropathic pain syndromes, including antidepressants, anticonvulsants and opioids. Many non-steroidal anti-inflammatory drugs are useful, and there is interest in the use of cyclooxygenase-2 inhibitors.

Antibiotics. There is currently no role for antibiotics in the management of PBS/IC in the absence of a laboratory-proven UTI.

TABLE 7.4

Tricyclic antidepressants used to treat interstitial cystitis

- Amitryptyline
- Imipramine
- Nortriptyline
- Desipramine
- Doxepin

Hydroxyzine is a histamine H_1 receptor antagonist that inhibits bladder mast-cell activation. It has been reported to reduce frequency, nocturia and pain in a small proportion of patients, but efficacy was not demonstrated in a double-blind randomized controlled trial.

Sodium pentosanpolysulfate is a heparin analog available in an oral formulation, 3–6% of which is excreted into the urine. Although this is the only oral agent approved for the treatment of IC, expert opinion of its efficacy is divided. As a sulfated mucopolysaccharide, sodium pentosanpolysulfate is hypothesized to repair defects in the glycoaminoglycan layer of the epithelial permeability barrier, which are thought to contribute to the pathogenesis of IC. It has been reported by advocates as beneficial in that it reduces the symptoms of IC to a modestly greater extent than placebo. A 3–6-month course is needed to demonstrate an effect; the dose is 100 mg three times a day. Sodium pentosanpolysulfate is well tolerated and produces few side effects.

Intravesical therapy. Several drugs are available for intravesical therapy of IC. These include chlorpactin, dimethyl sulfoxide (DMSO), heparin, hyaluronic acid and sodium pentosanpolysulfate.

The intravesical route of administration provides high local drug concentrations in the bladder, avoids systemic side effects and eliminates the problem of low levels of urinary excretion with orally administered agents. Agents are given weekly or every 2 weeks for a total of 4–8 treatments. Long-term remission will be achieved in some patients with this approach, but in most the condition will relapse eventually and require additional treatments.

Treatment with intravesical agents does not require anesthesia or hospital admission, and some patients can be taught to self-administer the drugs.

Invasive treatment should be reserved for patients with debilitating symptoms in whom conservative treatments have failed.

Sacral nerve stimulation (see Figure 4.2, pages 52–3) involves the percutaneous stimulation of the S3 or S4 nerve root. Initially it is carried out with a temporary stimulator; a permanent implant can be inserted if the patient responds.

Augmentation cystoplasty was used for refractory bladder pain for many years but is rarely used nowadays. The procedure involves using a segment of bowel to enlarge the bladder and has been performed with or without excision of the diseased bladder segment. However, results are generally poor for classic PBS/IC.

Key points – urinary tract infections and cystitis

- Recurrent urinary tract infection (UTI) is defined as a further UTI after resolution of initial bacteriuria.
- At least 20–30% of women will have a UTI at some time, 25% of whom will develop recurrent UTI. UTIs are relatively rare in men and are more likely to have a significant cause than in women.
- Urinalysis is quick and easy. A positive test should be followed up by microscopy, and the urine cultured to determine antimicrobial sensitivity.
- Treatment of UTIs is largely on the basis of symptoms and any underlying identified cause.
- Antibiotic treatment is recommended for recurrent UTI; prophylactic antibiotics and self-medication should also be considered.
- Painful bladder syndrome (PBS) is characterized by suprapubic pain relating to bladder filling, accompanied by other symptoms such as frequency, in the absence of a proven UTI or other pathology. The diagnosis of interstitial cystitis (IC) is confined to patients with painful bladder symptoms with characteristic cytoscopic and histological features.
- The etiology of PBS/IC is largely unknown.
- The roles of cystoscopy and bladder biopsy in the diagnosis of PBS/IC are controversial.
- Management of PBS/IC is largely conservative, and includes dietary advice, behavioral therapies, and oral and intravesical medication.

Key references

Albert X, Huertas I, Pereiró I et al. Antibiotics for preventing recurrent urinary tract infection in non-pregnant women. *Cochrane Database Syst Rev* 2004, issue 3. CD001209. www.thecochranelibrary.com

Franco AV. Recurrent urinary tract infections. *Best Pract Res Clin Obstet Gynaecol* 2005;19:861–73.

Hanno PM. Painful bladder syndrome / interstitial cystitis and related disorders. In: Wein AJ, Kavoussi LR, Novick AC et al., eds. *Campbell-Walsh Urology*. Philadelphia: Elsevier/Saunders, 2007:330–70.

Moldwin RM, Evans RJ, Stanford EJ, Rosenberg MT. Rational approaches to the treatment of patients with interstitial cystitis. *Urology* 2007;69(4 Suppl):73–81.

Rosenberg M, Parsons CL, Page S. Interstitial cystitis: a primary care perspective. *Cleve Clin J Med* 2005;72:698–704.

Primary nocturnal enuresis

Primary nocturnal enuresis is urinary incontinence that occurs during sleep in a child who has never regularly been dry at night. It is a common condition that can cause difficulty for both child and family. Nocturnal enuresis occurs in approximately 20% of 5-year-olds, 10% of 10-year-olds and 1% of 15-year-olds.

The majority of children affected are fully continent during the day. The condition is usually self-limiting and children generally become dry at night spontaneously as they get older.

Etiology. Nocturnal enuresis has a number of different etiologies:
- high fluid intake in association with heavy sleeping
- reduced urine osmolarity decreases nocturnal secretion of antidiuretic hormone (ADH; desmopressin), leading to increased night-time urine production
- detrusor overactivity, seen in 25% of children with nocturnal enuresis with no daytime symptoms
- upper airway obstruction is associated with nocturnal enuresis; the latter condition improves with treatment such as tonsillectomy
- family history, noted in 65–77% of children with nocturnal enuresis
- psychological factors, possibly (some disagreement).

Investigations. A comprehensive urologic history should be taken to exclude any associated conditions that may require treatment. Physical examination should be carried out, although abnormalities are unlikely to be detected. The specific gravity of an early-morning urine sample should be measured to identify those who may benefit from ADH (desmopressin) treatment.

A *urinary diary* (see Chapter 2, pages 20–1) is one of the most important tools in the investigation and management of primary nocturnal enuresis. It will provide detailed information about fluid intake and voided volumes during the day and episodes of bed-wetting during the night. It can be used to assess the severity of the problem and also provides a baseline against which the effects of treatment can be measured.

Renal ultrasound and uroflowmetry are required only when symptoms are suggestive of urinary tract dysfunction. Urodynamic studies should be reserved for patients with diurnal symptoms that fail to respond to conventional treatments.

Treatment. Many different treatments have been tried for nocturnal enuresis, with varying degrees of success. The success rates of common treatments are shown in Table 8.1.

Reassurance. The majority of children will grow out of bed-wetting, and reassurance may be all that is necessary. However, most parents and children ask for treatment because of the inconvenience and social difficulty that bed-wetting causes.

Changes in fluid intake and therefore output are the simplest means of improving the condition; keeping a diary is important to record improvements. It is important not to set a high and unattainable goal too early or the child will lose interest. Although parents are often tempted to control evening drinking, this may be counterproductive because concentrated urine can irritate the bladder.

Behavioral therapy. If the child wets the bed at a particular time of night, a waking regimen may be of benefit. Behavioral therapy and biofeedback are useful non-pharmacological treatments. Alarms that sense bed-wetting can be used from the age of 7 years, but become most effective after the age of 10 years when the child is able to take responsibility for him- or herself.

Pharmacological treatment. Antimuscarinic drugs (see Table 4.3, page 51) can be beneficial. ADH (desmopressin) will reduce nocturnal urine output and provide dry nights, but is not recommended for continuous long-term use because of alterations in serum electrolytes. However, it can be useful if a child is sleeping away from home.

Persistence into adolescence. Only 1% of adolescents (by age 15 years) still experience nocturnal enuresis, and 15% of these become dry with each subsequent year. By 15 years of age urodynamic studies should be performed to check for abnormalities in detrusor function, the commonest of these being detrusor overactivity. Occult neurological dysfunction may be responsible for enuresis in a small number of

TABLE 8.1

Efficacy of common treatments for nocturnal enuresis

Treatment	Efficacy
Observation only	• 6% continent at 6 months; 16% at 1 year
Drug therapy	
ADH (desmopressin)	• Improvement in 79% of patients at 1 year; 50% long-term improvement • 68% continent at 6 months; 10% continent at 1 year • 81% improved by 12 weeks • 48% dry and 22% improved
Amitriptyline	• Effective at reducing number of wet nights
Imipramine	• 36% continent at 6 months; 16% at 1 year; 73% improved
Behavioral interventions	
Alarms and sensors	• 84% dry • 63% continent at 6 months; 56% at 1 year
Waking schedule and full-spectrum home training	• 76% dry
Motivation counseling	• 23% cure rate (many more helped)
Acupuncture	• 55% effective at 1 year; 40% long-term improvement
Combination – drugs plus alarms	• May produce a complementary benefit

ADH, antidiuretic hormone.

patients. After the age of 18 years, patients with persistent enuresis due to detrusor overactivity that does not respond to non-surgical treatment could be offered treatment with botulinum toxin or bladder augmentation (see Chapter 4, pages 50 and 54, respectively).

Nocturia and nocturnal polyuria

Nocturia is defined as waking from sleep once or more to void, with each void preceded and followed by sleep. It is the lower urinary tract symptom that has the greatest impact on quality of life and is particularly prevalent in the elderly. It is often associated with nocturnal polyuria and is a common cause of falls when trying to reach the bathroom.

Etiology. Diuresis is normally reduced at night. In nocturnal polyuria, more than one-third of the 24-hour urine production occurs at night. This is frequently a result of dependent extravascular fluid re-entering the circulation when the lower limbs are elevated in bed, as a result of venous insufficiency and congestive cardiac failure.

Investigation. The urinary diary (see Chapter 2, pages 20–1) is the most useful tool for investigating nocturia: it will provide information about the number of night-time voids and fluid intake, particularly in the evening.

Urodynamic studies can be carried out to identify detrusor overactivity. If congestive cardiac failure is suspected, the appropriate investigations and referral should be made.

Treatment of nocturia should be on the basis of identified underlying causes. Simple measures can be implemented, such as reducing night-time fluid intake. The frail elderly should be provided with a bedside commode, to minimize the risk of falls while going to the bathroom. An upright rail fixed to the bed to facilitate getting out safely is also important.

Pharmacological treatment aims to shift the diuresis to the daytime. Reducing the volume overload associated with congestive cardiac failure with a dose of loop diuretic 6–8 hours before bed may be helpful.

ADH (desmopressin) has been used successfully to reduce nocturnal urine output. However, it can cause hyponatremia, and there is a risk of exacerbating congestive cardiac failure, particularly in the elderly; it is therefore not generally suitable for patients over 65 years of age. If treatment is commenced, it is important to measure serum electrolytes beforehand and 1–3 days after commencing treatment, as hyponatremia can develop rapidly.

A trial of antimuscarinics (see Table 4.3, page 51) is likely to be beneficial if the nocturia is associated with bladder filling/storage symptoms, particularly in younger patients.

Key points – nocturnal symptoms

- Primary nocturnal enuresis is urinary incontinence that occurs at night in a child who has never been regularly dry at night.
- It is a relatively common condition, but generally resolves spontaneously and rarely persists into adolescence.
- The urinary diary is the most useful investigative tool for primary nocturnal enuresis and also helps in monitoring treatment.
- Treatment of primary nocturnal enuresis is rarely required, but can include modification of fluid intake, behavioral treatments and occasional use of antidiuretic hormone (ADH; desmopressin).
- Nocturia – defined as waking from sleep to void – has a significant impact on quality of life and is a major cause of falls in the elderly.
- Treatment of nocturia is largely on the basis of the underlying cause. Loop diuretics in the afternoon may be useful if nocturia is related to congestive heart failure. ADH should be used with caution, as it can cause rapid hyponatremia. Antimuscarinics may prove useful in patients with overactive bladder.

Key references

Glazener CMA, Evans JHC. Desmopressin for nocturnal enuresis in children. *Cochrane Database Syst Rev* 2002, issue 3. CD002112. www.thecochranelibrary.com

Glazener CMA, Evans JHC. Simple behavioural and physical interventions for nocturnal enuresis in children. *Cochrane Database Syst Rev* 2004, issue 2. CD003637. www.thecochranelibrary.com

Glazener CMA, Evans JHC, Peto RE. Drugs for nocturnal enuresis in children (other than desmopressin and tricyclics). *Cochrane Database Syst Rev* 2003, issue 4. CD002238. www.thecochranelibrary.com

Lyon C, Schnall J. What is the best treatment for nocturnal enuresis in children? *J Fam Pract* 2005;54: 905–6, 909.

Most neurological diseases that affect the spinal cord and some that affect the brain will cause bladder dysfunction, which, if untreated, may lead to incontinence. Neuropathic bladder dysfunction can be divided into three types of disorder according to the site of the lesion: suprapontine, suprasacral spinal and peripheral. Urodynamic investigation is required to distinguish between the different types of filling/storage and voiding dysfunction that may result.

Suprapontine lesions tend to lead to detrusor overactivity, although coordinated sphincter function is preserved. These lesions can therefore result in frequency, urgency and urge incontinence. The principal causes of suprapontine lesions are dementia, cerebrovascular accident and Parkinson's disease.

Suprasacral spinal lesions that interfere with reflex control of the bladder from the higher centers will produce detrusor overactivity. This is seen in many patients with neurological bladder dysfunction and is characterized by spontaneous involuntary detrusor contractions, with or without the sensation of urgency, leading to urinary incontinence. Detrusor overactivity may be associated with non-coordination of the external urethral sphincter, which contracts during detrusor contraction, termed detrusor–sphincter dyssynergia (DSD). This causes hypertrophy of detrusor smooth muscle (trabeculation) as a result of the frequent, high-pressure, sustained detrusor contractions in the presence of obstruction. Patients with detrusor overactivity and DSD not only experience urinary incontinence but may also develop long-term effects of high intravesical pressures, giving rise to ureteric reflux or obstruction, or both, and resulting in renal damage and failure.

The causes of suprasacral spinal lesions include multiple sclerosis, Parkinson's disease, spinal cord injury, spina bifida and tumors that affect the suprasacral spinal cord.

Peripheral lesions. Injury or disease that affects the nerve roots or peripheral nerves (spinal trauma, pelvic surgery, diabetes mellitus) causes bladder areflexia or acontractility and, as a result, the bladder fails to empty unless voiding is assisted by straining. In patients with such lesions, the external urethral sphincter may fail to relax (isolated distal sphincter obstruction) and may also be weakened, giving rise to sphincter weakness incontinence.

Diagnosis

The diagnosis of neuropathic bladder disorders requires an understanding of the underlying neurological abnormality, which will be apparent in most patients. However, some patients will present with the symptoms of a neuropathic bladder but with no overt neurological cause. In this situation it is important to consider the possibility of an undiagnosed neurological condition such as multiple sclerosis or spinal cord lesion, as neuropathic bladder may be the presenting symptom. In patients with cervical lesions, especially those with complete spinal cord transection, it may be difficult to assess symptoms as many will be atypical or unconscious rather than the classic 'urge' type symptoms.

Patients with acontractile bladders tend to leak urine as a result of retention with overflow or in association with sphincter weakness.

Apart from neurological examination, urodynamic investigation is essential to make an appropriate diagnosis and provide treatment.

Management

The aim of treating the neuropathic bladder is to enable low-pressure storage of urine and bladder emptying without obstruction. Treatment is therefore focused on reducing detrusor muscle contractions and/or reducing the effect of DSD by lowering the resistance of the external urethral sphincter.

Control of detrusor overactivity with antimuscarinic drugs or surgery is described in Chapter 4 (pages 49–50 and 54–5, respectively). If oral therapy cannot be tolerated, intravesical agents such as botulinum toxin or oxybutynin may be used.

Reducing resistance in the external urethral sphincter can be achieved by a number of methods: sphincterotomy, sphincter stenting or injection of botulinum toxin. These procedures are only suitable for men, who should be counseled about the risk of continuous incontinence afterwards.

In women, a reduction in detrusor contractility will often lead to urinary retention, and intermittent self-catheterization may be necessary to drain the bladder fully (see below).

Sphincter weakness incontinence, which accompanies neurological bladder dysfunction, may be resolved by procedures to enhance the bladder outlet (see Chapter 3, pages 42–5).

Catheterization. Despite these measures, some patients will continue to have problems with DSD and will require catheterization to empty the bladder and prevent the long-term complications associated with the condition. The options for these patients are clean intermittent self-catheterization, or long-term catheterization with a urethral or suprapubic catheter.

Clean intermittent self-catheterization (Figure 9.1) is useful in any condition in which bladder emptying is impaired in association with adequate outlet resistance. It is used instead of normal bladder emptying on a regular basis throughout the day (and night). The number of catheterizations required will depend on factors such as fluid intake, ambient temperature, bladder capacity and social factors; most patients need to empty the bladder four or five times each day.

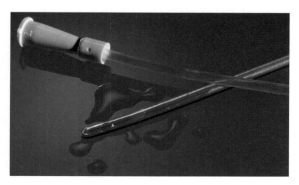

Figure 9.1
Special catheters are used for clean intermittent self-catheterization

For self-catheterization to be successful in patients with neuropathic bladder dysfunction, the bladder must be able to store urine adequately without leaking, a condition that can be facilitated through the use of antimuscarinic medication (see Table 4.3, page 51). The patient must be physically able and motivated to perform catheterization, or a caregiver must be able to do it for them. Patients and caregivers need access to health professionals who can teach them the technique and provide adequate support and suitable catheters.

Long-term (permanent) catheterization is usually a last resort when all other treatments have failed. However, it may occasionally be used for shorter periods if patients are undecided about their preferred management option. For long-term catheterization, the suprapubic catheter avoids urethral damage, and is more comfortable and better tolerated than a catheter inserted via the urethra. It is also easier to change on a regular basis and causes less discomfort than may be experienced when changing a urethral catheter.

Insertion of a suprapubic catheter should be carried out under ultrasound or cystoscopic guidance, as there is a risk of bowel trauma from incorrect placement of the catheter. Mortality associated with insertion has been reported as being up to 2%.

Catheter changes. In general, most all-silicone catheters need to be changed every 6–8 weeks. The catheter should be changed by an appropriately trained person, who can be a doctor, nurse, caregiver, relative or the patient.

Catheter problems. If a suprapubic catheter falls out it is important that it is replaced quickly, ideally immediately. The tract will start to close extremely quickly and after 2 hours it is usually impossible to reinsert the catheter without dilatation of the tract. It is therefore essential that the patient is transferred to hospital immediately if no one is available to insert a replacement catheter. Patients should keep a spare catheter at home in case problems arise.

Catheter blockage is a common problem, usually occurring as a result of calcification or the accumulation of debris. Some patients are more prone to catheter blockage than others. If blockage occurs on a regular basis, imaging and/or cystoscopy should be performed to look for bladder calculi or other abnormalities. If investigation suggests calculi, cystoscopy should be performed and the stones removed. Patients who frequently have blocked catheters should be managed with high fluid intake and more regular catheter changes.

Follow-up. All patients with spinal cord injury and bladder dysfunction are susceptible to renal damage if the intravesical pressure is not adequately controlled. Yearly follow-up with at least ultrasonography of the upper urinary tracts and measurement of serum creatinine is therefore essential.

Key points – neuropathic bladder dysfunction

- Neuropathic bladder dysfunction can be classified according to the site of the lesion as suprapontine, suprasacral spinal or peripheral.
- Suprapontine lesions are largely associated with Parkinson's disease, dementia and cerebrovascular accident. They usually lead to detrusor overactivity but coordinated sphincter function is preserved.
- Suprasacral spinal lesions are associated with spinal cord injury, spina bifida and tumors, and interfere with the reflex control of the bladder from higher centers, resulting in detrusor overactivity and detrusor–sphincter dyssynergia. Increased intravesical pressure can damage the ureters and, ultimately, the kidneys.
- Peripheral lesions affecting the nerve roots cause bladder areflexia or acontractility, such that the bladder fails to empty without straining. Sphincteric weakness may also contribute to incontinence.
- Management aims to enable low-pressure storage of urine and bladder emptying without obstruction, achieved by antimuscarinic drugs, injection of botulinum toxin or surgery.
- Some patients require catheterization to ensure bladder emptying. Options are clean intermittent self-catheterization, if the bladder can store urine adequately without leaking (often achieved with antimuscarinic drugs), or a permanent urethral or suprapubic catheter.

Key references

Bray L, Sanders C. Teaching children and young people intermittent self-catheterization. *Urol Nurs* 2007;27:203–9, 242.

Rapidi CA, Panourias IG, Petropoulou K, Sakas DE. Management and rehabilitation of neuropathic bladder in patients with spinal cord lesion. *Acta Neurochir Suppl* 2007;97:307–14.

Samson G, Cardenas DD. Neurogenic bladder in spinal cord injury. *Phys Med Rehabil Clin N Am* 2007;18:255–74.

Stöhrer M, Castro-Diaz D, Chartier-Kastler E et al. Guidelines on neurogenic lower urinary tract dysfunction. European Association of Urology, 2003. www.uroweb.org/fileadmin/user _upload/Guidelines/neurogenic.pdf

Wein AJ. Lower urinary tract dysfunction in neurologic injury and disease. In: Wein AJ, Kavoussi LR, Novick AC et al., eds. *Campbell-Walsh Urology*. Philadelphia: Elsevier/Saunders, 2007:2011–45.

The elderly

Lower urinary tract symptoms become more prevalent with age. Management of the symptoms can be challenging, as the elderly are less likely to tolerate surgical or pharmaceutical treatments and their symptoms are often secondary to multiple causes.

The approach to treatment of these symptoms in the elderly is similar to that in younger people, as the underlying pathophysiology of incontinence does not differ markedly. It is important to rule out or treat constipation, urinary tract infection (UTI) and inappropriate medication before embarking on extensive investigation.

Urinary incontinence is a frequent cause of institutionalization in the elderly. The common causes of incontinence are similar to those found in younger people, namely bladder overactivity and sphincter weakness, but the effects of aging on the nervous system and the lower urinary tract exacerbate the symptoms.

As in younger people, it is appropriate to determine the cause of incontinence and it is feasible to correct both bladder overactivity and sphincter weakness.

Investigation. Finding the cause of urinary incontinence is more important in the elderly than in younger patients. The elderly are more likely to have multiple coexisting symptoms and may have multiple pathologies to account for them. In addition, the elderly are less likely to tolerate the adverse effects of antimuscarinic medications, and these drugs are more likely to precipitate urinary retention. Empirical treatment based on symptoms and a urinary diary is therefore unsatisfactory.

Investigation may involve urodynamic investigation, the indications for which are outlined in Chapter 2. Cystometry is well tolerated in the elderly. If cystometry is performed, prophylactic antibiotics should be considered, particularly in patients susceptible to UTIs.

Treatment. If detrusor overactivity is identified, behavioral modification and antimuscarinic medication can be commenced, taking into account other medications the patient is taking that may cause interactions, such as antidepressants. Treatment should be started with a low dose and the dose increased gradually until the required benefits are obtained with the minimum of adverse effects. Detrusor contractility decreases with age and therefore the incidence of urinary retention with antimuscarinic medications is higher in the elderly.

In women, urethral hypermobility becomes a less prevalent cause of urinary stress incontinence with age as vaginal mobility reduces with postmenopausal atrophy. This means that stress incontinence is far more likely to be secondary to intrinsic sphincter deficiency in these patients, and treatment should be tailored accordingly.

Surgery for stress incontinence is possible in the elderly but general anesthesia and major abdominal surgery are best avoided. Urethral injection therapy or minimally invasive sling insertion under local or regional anesthesia (as described in Chapter 3) are well tolerated.

The risk of postoperative urinary retention is relatively high in the elderly because of their reduced detrusor contractility. Retention is also more difficult to manage, as intermittent self-catheterization can be impossible in those with poor eyesight and reduced manual dexterity.

Urethral injection therapy is preferred in the frail elderly; although efficacy is lower than in younger patients, the incidence of postoperative retention is also reduced.

Urinary frequency and nocturia. As the bladder ages, its functional capacity decreases and filling symptoms such as urgency and frequency become more prevalent. Nocturia is particularly common in the elderly and is discussed in Chapter 8. Bladder filling symptoms may be secondary to detrusor overactivity; however, intravesical pathologies such as interstitial cystitis and tumors are more likely than in younger patients and further investigation with urine culture, cytology, urodynamic studies and cystoscopy may be required.

Voiding dysfunction. Poor detrusor contractility is common in the elderly and can impair voiding even in the absence of bladder outlet obstruction. Urinary retention may follow, which, if chronic, may be painless but can lead to overflow incontinence. It is also common for factors such as constipation, medication (such as antimuscarinics and α-adrenergic agonists) and bed rest to unmask subclinical voiding dysfunction and lead to retention.

Neurological problems can lead to voiding dysfunction. These include spinal cord compression resulting from a tumor or vertebral collapse, stroke, sensory loss and Parkinson's disease. Stroke may initially cause retention, which is replaced by neurogenic detrusor overactivity. Parkinson's disease results in voiding dysfunction, primarily as a result of detrusor overactivity, bradykinesia of the striated sphincter or poor detrusor contractility. Sensory loss is most commonly caused by diabetes; it may lead to progressive bladder distension, voiding dysfunction and acontractility, resulting in overflow incontinence.

Urinary retention. The aims of initial management are to stop any implicated factors such as medication and to rectify any reversible factors, such as prolapse in women. If this fails then the treatment of choice is self-catheterization. However, this may not be feasible for the reasons outlined above, and long-term suprapubic catheterization may be the only option.

Urinary tract infections are common in elderly women, occurring in up to 46% of long-stay geriatric patients over the course of a year. This is normally the result of multiple factors, such as impaired immunology, voiding dysfunction and urinary stasis, genital atrophy, fecal incontinence and low fluid intake. There is also an increased likelihood of intravesical pathology. Investigation with flexible cystoscopy is recommended in the case of recurrent UTIs.

Treatment of UTIs in elderly women with no identifiable pathology is with low-dose vaginal estrogen and prophylactic antibiotics, as described in Chapter 7.

Polypharmacy (the use of multiple medications concurrently) is common in the elderly, and incontinence is frequently a result of medications prescribed for other conditions. Drugs can adversely affect bladder function in a number of ways, summarized in Table 10.1.

TABLE 10.1

Adverse effects of drugs on bladder function

Increased diuresis	• Diuretic medications and alcohol increase the rate of bladder filling and aggravate lower urinary tract symptoms
Decreased detrusor contractility	• Antimuscarinics, α-adrenergic agonists and calcium-channel blockers can decrease bladder contractility, and can precipitate urinary retention and subsequent overflow incontinence in a patient with poor intrinsic detrusor function
Alterations in urethral tone	• α-adrenoceptors may be responsible for the urethral sphincter tone; any medications that act as α-adrenergic agonists may therefore precipitate urinary retention, and antagonists may aggravate incontinence
	• β-adrenergic agonists, particularly β-2 agonists, and benzodiazepines can cause muscle relaxation and exacerbate urinary stress incontinence

Pregnancy

Lower urinary tract symptoms are common during pregnancy, and childbirth is often cited as a cause for subsequent urinary, colorectal and genital dysfunction. The hormonal effects of pregnancy also can be responsible for other urinary tract pathology such as hydronephrosis and UTIs.

Bladder filling symptoms

Frequency. Between 45% and 90% of women will develop urinary frequency as pregnancy progresses. This is the result of increased renal blood flow, which increases urine production, and compression of the bladder by the enlarging uterus.

Urgency is a common symptom in pregnancy, reported by up to 70% of women. It has been proposed that high progesterone levels may be the cause of detrusor overactivity in pregnancy, although urodynamic findings show detrusor overactivity in only approximately 25% of women who complain of urge incontinence in pregnancy.

Antimuscarinic medication is contraindicated in pregnancy, so management is limited to bladder training, physiotherapy and restriction of caffeine intake.

Nocturia is common in pregnancy and is rarely pathological. It is caused by increased urine production and mobilization of dependent edema when the legs are elevated during sleep.

Urinary incontinence. Stress urinary incontinence in pregnancy is common – it has been reported in up to 85% of pregnant women. It is likely to be caused by pressure from the pregnant uterus, combined with relaxation of the pelvic ligaments and smooth musculature in response to the high levels of progesterone and other pregnancy hormones.

Prenatal stress incontinence usually resolves spontaneously after delivery, and the mainstay of treatment is physiotherapy and supervised pelvic floor exercises (see Box 3.1, page 37).

Intrapartum risk factors. A number of intrapartum events have been shown to contribute to postnatal urinary stress incontinence. Vaginal delivery, particularly in association with a prolonged second stage, assisted delivery, high birth weight and third-degree perineal tears can damage the pelvic floor innervation and increase pudendal nerve latency. Delivery with forceps appears to be associated with a higher incidence of stress incontinence than vacuum extraction and unassisted delivery.

While there is a widely held belief that cesarean section protects against postpartum incontinence, the link is controversial and the evidence around it is conflicting. A prospective study of 1169 women undergoing elective cesarean section showed that although the incidence of incontinence was reduced at 6 months postpartum, cesarean section did not prevent incontinence.

It therefore seems likely that both pregnancy and delivery can cause pelvic floor dysfunction.

Voiding symptoms

During pregnancy. One-third of women report hesitancy and incomplete bladder emptying during pregnancy, but these symptoms are rarely associated with voiding disorders on urodynamic testing.

Urinary retention occurs occasionally, usually in association with entrapment of a retroverted uterus in the second trimester. Management involves bladder drainage and manual reduction of the uterus. If retroversion recurs, a pessary can be inserted temporarily to keep the uterus in the anteverted position, relieving the obstruction on the bladder neck.

Postnatal disorders. The most common cause of postnatal voiding disorders and urinary retention is the use of epidural and spinal anesthesia during labor and delivery. However, all women are at risk of urinary retention, and careful surveillance during and after delivery is important. Urinary retention requires prompt catheterization. It should be noted that many women have reduced bladder sensation after delivery, and urinary retention may not present with pain. Failure to recognize and manage postpartum urinary retention risks long-term bladder damage as a result of overdistension, denervation and atony of the detrusor muscle, which may require long-term catheterization.

Hydronephrosis is a common finding in pregnancy and is related to smooth muscle relaxation and the pressure of the enlarged uterus. It is more common on the right side. Hydronephrosis is largely asymptomatic and does not require treatment, and will resolve spontaneously on delivery.

If a woman presents with pain secondary to hydronephrosis, analgesia is usually all that is required. In the rare cases of renal impairment secondary to obstruction, ureteric stenting or percutaneous nephrostomy under radiological guidance is indicated.

Urinary tract infections. The smooth muscle relaxation associated with high levels of progesterone in pregnancy may predispose women to UTIs by affecting bladder emptying and ureteric drainage. UTIs are known to be associated with preterm delivery and low birth weight, so screening for infection and administering correct treatment are important.

Asymptomatic bacteriuria refers to the finding of more than 105 colony forming units (CFU) per mL urine, which develops into pyelonephritis in 20–40% of pregnant women if left untreated, but only 1–2% if treated adequately.

Pregnant women should be screened for UTI at all antenatal visits; if a UTI has been treated, the patient should be followed up closely for signs of recurrence. If recurrent UTIs occur, then appropriate low-dose prophylactic antibiotics may be used until delivery.

Fistula-related incontinence

A fistula is an abnormal communication between two epithelialized structures. The urinary tract fistula most commonly responsible for urinary incontinence is the vesicovaginal fistula (VVF; Figure 10.1).

Etiology of VVF differs in various parts of the world. In developed countries, 75% of cases are iatrogenic, caused by injury to the bladder at the time of pelvic or gynecologic surgery. Obstetric trauma accounts for very few cases of VVF in developed countries, but is still a common

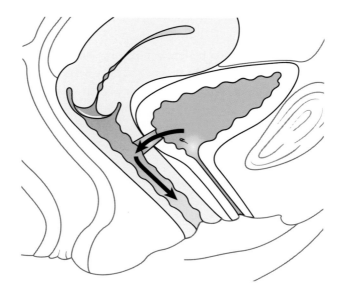

Figure 10.1 A vesicovaginal fistula.

cause in developing countries as a result of prolonged unsupervised labor. Other causes of VVF include pelvic malignancy, radiotherapy, trauma and gynecologic/urologic instrumentation.

Diagnosis. A woman with a VVF will commonly complain of continuous drainage of urine from the vagina, although small fistulas can present with intermittent leakage that is positional in nature. If the fistula is large, the patient may not void normally at all and may have continuous leakage of urine into the vagina.

A VVF that has occurred after surgery commonly presents upon removal of the urethral catheter or up to 3 weeks later with urinary drainage from the vagina. VVF caused by radiation therapy may present many months or even years after completion of radiotherapy.

It is important to distinguish VVF from other causes of urinary incontinence; investigations should include a full examination. If a fistula is suspected but is not identified on examination with a Sims' speculum, further investigations will be needed to make the diagnosis. Even when the diagnosis can be made clinically, investigation may be needed to plan treatment.

Investigations

Examination under anesthesia may be required to determine the presence of a fistula. It is also important to assess the mobility of the tissues and the accessibility of a fistula for surgical repair.

Cystoscopy may also be carried out as part of this investigation. Although there is some debate as to the role of cystoscopy in the management of fistulas, it does enable the exact level of the fistula and its relation to the ureteric orifices and bladder neck to be assessed. In addition, a biopsy should be performed of the edge of any fistula that is related to radiotherapy or thought to be malignant.

Dye studies. The site of a fistula can be identified by instilling methylene blue dye into the bladder via a catheter, with the patient in the lithotomy position. The vagina is then inspected and the presence of fistulous communications noted. If urine continues to leak into the vagina despite a negative dye test, a ureteric fistula must be suspected.

Intravenous urography (IVU) should be performed in all cases of suspected urinary tract fistula. Although IVU is not particularly sensitive in the diagnosis of VVF, knowledge of the upper urinary tracts may be important when considering treatment. Ureteric dilatation is commonly seen with ureteric fistulas; if it is found in association with a known VVF then a complex fistula should be suspected.

Retrograde pyeloureterography is useful to identify the exact site of a ureteric fistula or to definitely rule one out, and can be undertaken at the same time as therapeutic stenting of the ureter.

Treatment

Conservative management. The initial management of most urinary tract fistulas is conservative. VVFs may heal spontaneously with continuous bladder drainage over a period of 6–8 weeks, and a ureterovaginal fistula may resolve if the affected ureter is stented for 6–12 weeks. During the period of conservative management, the patient should be provided with incontinence pads and with barrier cream to protect the vulval skin, which is at risk of dermatitis as a result of prolonged contact with urine.

Surgical management. There is some debate as to the timing of surgical treatment of urinary tract fistulas. Early treatment is advocated by some because of the social and psychological benefits to women who are already distressed. However, most fistulas are associated with tissue inflammation and sloughing, and success rates are reduced if surgery is performed before this has resolved. It is therefore important not to be pressured by the patient into operating on a fistula too soon, as this may jeopardize the surgical outcome.

Fistulas can be repaired vaginally or abdominally; the principle of repair is the same for both routes. The fistula is identified and its tract excised. The layers are then closed. Success can be enhanced by interposition of healthy tissue between the bladder and vagina to create an additional layer to the repair. Tissues commonly used are omentum or a Martius graft of labial fat and bulbocavernosus muscle passed subcutaneously to cover the repair.

Key points – special considerations

- The prevalence of urinary tract symptoms increases with age, and urinary incontinence is a frequent cause of institutionalization of the elderly.
- Identification of the cause is more important in the elderly than in younger patients, as elderly patients are likely to have multiple coexisting symptoms and pathologies. Polypharmacy may be a contributory factor.
- Urinary tract infection (UTI) is common in elderly women. Treatment of persistent UTI is with low-dose vaginal estrogen and prophylactic antibiotics.
- Lower urinary tract problems are common in pregnancy and usually resolve after delivery.
- Vaginal delivery, especially associated with a long second stage of labor, forceps-assisted delivery and high birth weight, may damage the pelvic floor innervation and result in postnatal incontinence.
- UTIs are common in pregnancy and are associated with preterm delivery and low birth weight. Pregnant women should therefore be screened for UTIs at all antenatal visits, and UTIs treated accordingly.
- Vesicovaginal fistula (VVF), which results in vaginal leakage of urine, is the most common fistula to cause urinary incontinence.
- In developed countries VVF may be caused by pelvic malignancy, radiotherapy, trauma and gynecologic/urologic instrumentation. Obstetric trauma during unsupervised labor is a common cause of VVF in developing countries.
- Dye studies and imaging are required to determine the site of a fistula.
- Many fistulas heal spontaneously over 6–12 weeks with conservative management such as bladder draining or ureteric stenting. Premature surgery is likely to be unsuccessful because of tissue inflammation and sloughing.

Key references

FitzGerald MP, Graziano S. Anatomic and functional changes of the lower urinary tract during pregnancy. *Urol Clin North Am* 2007;34:7–12.

Genadry R. A urogynecologist's view of the pelvic floor effects of vaginal delivery/cesarean section for the urologist. *Curr Urol Rep* 2006;7:376–83.

Wagg AS, Cardozo L, Chapple C et al. Overactive bladder syndrome in older people. *BJU Int* 2007;99: 502–9.

Wall LL. Obstetric vesicovaginal fistula as an international public-health problem. *Lancet* 2006;368:1201–9. www.endfistula.org/

Useful addresses

UK
Association for Continence Advice
c/o Fitwise Management Ltd
Drumcross Hall, Bathgate
West Lothian EH48 4JT
Tel: +44 (0)1506 811077
Fax: +44 (0)1506 811477
aca@fitwise.co.uk
www.aca.uk.com

British Association of Urological Surgeons
35–43 Lincoln's Inn Fields
London WC2A 3PE
Tel: +44 (0)20 7869 6950
Fax: +44 (0)20 7404 5048
admin@baus.org.uk
www.baus.org.uk

The Continence Foundation
307 Hatton Square
16 Baldwins Gardens
London ECIN 7RJ
Helpline: 0845 345 0165
(Mon–Fri 9.30 AM–1 PM)
Tel: +44 (0)20 7404 6875
Fax: +44 (0)20 7404 6876
continence-help@dial.pipex.com
www.continence-foundation.org.uk

The Cystitis and Overactive Bladder Foundation
76 High Street
Stony Stratford
Bucks MK11 1AH
Tel: +44 (0)1908 569169
Fax: +44 (0)1908 565665
info@cobfoundation.org
www.cobfoundation.org

ERIC (Education and Resources for Improving Childhood Continence)
34 Old School House
Britannia Road, Kingswood
Bristol BS15 8DB
Helpline: 0845 370 8008
(Mon–Fri 10 AM–4 PM)
Fax: +44 (0)117 960 0401
info@eric.org.uk
www.eric.org.uk

Incontact
(support and information for people with bladder and bowel problems)
SATRA Innovation Park
Rockingham Road
Kettering
Northants NN16 9JH
Tel: 0870 770 3246
Fax: 0870 770 3249
info@incontact.org
www.incontact.org

PromoCon

(product information, advice and practical solutions for people with continence difficulties)

Redbank House

4 St Chads Street, Cheetham

Manchester M8 8QA

Tel: 08707 601580

Fax: +44 (0)161 214 5961

Promocon@disabledliving.co.uk

www.promocon.co.uk

USA

American Academy of Family Physicians

PO Box 11210, Shawnee Mission

KS 66207-1210

Toll-free: 1 800 274 2237

Tel: +1 913 906 6000

fp@aafp.org

www.aafp.org

American Urological Association

1000 Corporate Boulevard

Linthicum, MD 21090

Toll-free: 1 866 746 4282

Tel: +1 410 689 3700

Fax: +1 410 689 3800

aua@auanet.org (general enquiries)

www.auanet.org

National Kidney Foundation

30 East 33rd Street

New York, NY 10016

Toll-free: 1 800 622 9010

Tel: +1 212 889 2210

Fax: +1 212 689 9261

www.kidney.org

Urology Channel

(comprehensive, physician-monitored information about urologic conditions)

www.urologychannel.com

International

Canadian Paediatric Society

www.caringforkids.cps.ca/behaviour/Bedwetting.htm

European Association of Urology

PO Box 30016

NL-6803 AA Arnhem

The Netherlands

Tel: +31 (0)26 389 0680

Fax: +31 (0)26 389 0674

www.uroweb.org

International Continence Society

19 Portland Square

Bristol BS2 8SJ

Tel: +44 (0)117 944 4881

Fax: +44 (0)117 944 4882

info@icsoffice.org

www.icsoffice.org

Index

abdominal examination 17
acupuncture 49
ADH *see* desmopressin
adolescence 83–5
α-1 adrenergic agonists 97
α-1 adrenoceptor antagonists 60
β-1 adrenergic agonists 97
ambulatory urodynamic investigation 29
analgesics 78
antibiotics 74–5, 78
antidepressants *see* serotonin and norepinephrine reuptake inhibitors; tricyclic antidepressants
antidiuretic hormone *see* desmopressin
antimuscarinics 49–50, 51, 83, 86, 94–5
artificial urinary sphincter 44–5
assessment, principles 14–30
augmentation cystoplasty 54–5, 79–80

bacteriology, UTI 72
bacteriuria, asymptomatic 71
  pregnancy 100
behavioral therapy 48–9, 78, 83, 84
biochemical tests *see* urinalysis
biofeedback training 35
biopsy 76
bladder
  capacity, evaluation 26
  catheterization 42, 90–2
  emptying *see* voiding
  neuropathic *see* neurological disease
bladder neck
  obstruction 57–8, 60–1, 62
  transurethral incision of prostate and 61

bladder outlet
  obstruction 56–60
  opening 11
  underactivity 31
bladder training 48–9, 78
botulinum toxin 50–1
brain lesions 88
bulking agents, injectable 41–2, 43, 95

caffeine intake reduction 35, 47
cancer *see* malignancy
carcinoma, transitional cell, cytology 66
catheterization 42, 90–2
  see also self-catheterization
central nervous system lesions 88
cesarean section 33, 98
childhood nocturnal enuresis 15, 82–5
colposuspension 39–41
complementary therapies 49
compliance, assessment 28
computed tomography 22, 68
congenital causes of bladder outlet obstruction 57
continence 9, 11
  loss of *see* incontinence
cranberry juice 74
cultures 20, 65
cystitis, interstitial 75–80
cystometry 24–8
cystoplasty *see* augmentation cystoplasty
cystoscopy 68, 76
cystourethroscopy, diagnostic 29
cytology, hematuria 66

darifenacin 51
delivery and stress incontinence 33–4, 98
desmopressin (ADH) 83, 84, 86

detrusor
  contractility 95–6, 97
  function, assessment 28
  myomectomy 55
  overactivity 23–4, 27, 42, 46, 49–50, 54–5, 82, 85, 88, 89, 94–5, 96
  pressure measurement 26–8
detrusor–sphincter dyssynergia 88, 89, 90
diary, urinary *see* frequency/volume chart
dietary management
  overactive bladder 47
  PBS/IC 77–8
  UTI 74
digital rectal examination 17, 58, 59
dipstick tests 20, 64, 73
diuresis, drug-induced 97
dribble
  postmicturition/postvoid 16, 31
  terminal 16
drug-induced conditions 64, 96, 97
drug treatment
  benign prostatic obstruction 60
  female stress incontinence 37
  incontinence in the elderly 94–5
  nocturnal enuresis 83, 84
  nocturnal polyuria/nocturia 85–6
  overactive bladder 49–51
  PBS/IC 77, 78–9
duloxetine hydrochloride 37

elderly 94–6
electrical nerve stimulation *see* neuromodulation
enuresis, nocturnal 15, 82–5
estrogen 32, 75
examination, principles 16–17

female/women
  genital examination 17
  incontinence 18, 32, 33–4,
    35–42, 95, 98, 100–1
  urinary tract anatomy 10
  UTI susceptibility 71
filling (urine storage) 10, 11,
  12
  symptoms 14–15, 97–8
filling cystometry 26–8
fistula-related incontinence
  100–2
fluid intake management 47,
  74, 83
follow-up 70, 92
frequency 14–15, 95
  night-time see nocturia
frequency/volume chart
  (urinary diary) 20, 21,
  46–7, 82–3, 85

genital examination 17

hematuria 64–70
hesitancy 16
history taking 14–16
hydronephrosis 57, 68, 99
hydroxyzine 77, 79

IC see interstitial cystitis
imaging 22, 68, 73, 102
  see also specific modalities
incomplete emptying 16
incontinence (urinary) 15,
  31–45
  assessment of 15, 20
  classification 31
  continuous 15
  definitions 31–2
  elderly 94–5
  fistula-related 100–2
  mixed 15, 32
  quality of life 18, 32
  risk factors 32, 33–4, 98
  stress see stress incontinence
  surgery see surgery
infections, urinary tract
  71–81
  elderly 96
  pregnancy 99–100
  recurrent 71–5

intermittent self-
  catheterization see self-
  catheterization
intermittent stream 16
international consultation on
  incontinence modular
  questionnaire (ICIQ) 18, 19
interstitial cystitis 75–80
intravenous urography 22,
  68, 102
intravesical drug therapy 79
investigations, principles
  18–24

kidney/renal tract (in
  hematuria)
  imaging 68, 83
  management of various
    pathologies 69
  pregnancy-related problems
    99

laboratory values see
  urinalysis
laser ablation of prostate 61
lifestyle changes 35, 47–8

male/men
  genital examination 17
  incontinence 18, 32, 34,
    42–5
  urinary tract anatomy 10
malignancy 64, 66
men see male/men
menopause and incontinence
  34
microbiology, UTI 72
microflora, vaginal 72
microscopy, hematuria 65
micturition see voiding
mid-urethral sling 38–9
minimally invasive surgery
  for stress incontinence,
  38–9, 43
muscarinic antagonists see
  antimuscarinics
myomectomy, detrusor 55

neoplasms see tumors
nerve stimulation, electrical
  see neuromodulation

neurological control of
  bladder function 9–10, 11
neurological disease
  (neuropathic bladder)
  88–93, 96
  urodynamic studies 24
neurological examination
  16–17
neuromodulation (incl.
  electrical nerve stimulation)
  35, 52, 79
neuropathic bladder see
  neurological disease
nocturia 15, 85–6
  elderly 95
  frequency/volume chart
    (urinary diary) 20, 85
  pregnancy 98
nocturnal enuresis 15,
  82–5
nocturnal polyuria 85–6
  frequency/volume chart
    (urinary diary) 20, 85

obstetrics see pregnancy
older people 94–6
one-stop clinics, hematuria
  68–9
overactive bladder 40–55
  detrusor overactivity
    compared with 46
  etiology 31, 46
  investigation 46–7
  management 47–55
oxybutynin 50, 51

painful bladder syndrome
  75–80
PBS see painful bladder
  syndrome
pelvic floor muscles 36
  assessment 17
  exercises for 35, 37
perineal sling 43
peripheral nervous system
  lesions 89
pharmacotherapy see drug
  treatment
physical examination,
  principles 16–17
plain films see radiography

polypharmacy, elderly 96
polyuria
  frequency/volume chart 20
  nocturnal *see* nocturnal
  polyuria
posterior urethral valves 57,
  58
postnatal voiding symptoms
  99
postvoid (postmicturition)
  dribble 16, 31
  residual volume,
  measurement 60
pregnancy 97–100
  incontinence and 33–4, 98,
  100–1
pressure flow studies 28
pressure measurements 26, 28
propiverine 51
prostate
  benign hyperplasia 56, 58,
  60–1
  digital rectal examination
  17, 58, 59
prostate-specific antigen
  (PSA) measurement 59
prostatectomy 34, 42–3, 44,
  61
proteinuria 65
psychological examination 18
pudendal nerve stimulation
  see transvaginal electrical
  stimulation
pyeloureterography,
  retrograde 102

quality of life 18, 19, 32

radiography 22, 69
radiology *see* imaging *and
  specific modalities*
reassurance, nocturnal
  enuresis 83
5α-reductase inhibitors 60
renal tract *see* kidney
reproductive hormones and
  incontinence 32
residual volume, postvoid,
  measurement 60
retrograde
  pyeloureterography 102

sacral nerve stimulation 52,
  53, 79
self-catheterization,
  intermittent 90–1
  neuropathic bladder 90–1
  stress incontinence surgery,
  postoperative 42
  UTI 73
sensation during filling,
  evaluation 26
serotonin and norepinephrine
  reuptake inhibitors, stress
  incontinence 37
sex (reproductive) hormones
  and incontinence 32
sling
  mid-urethral 38–9
  perineal 43
slow stream 16
sodium pentosanpolysulfate
  79
solifenacin 51
sphincter (external urethral)
  function 11
  incontinence related (men)
  42–5
  reducing resistance in 89,
  90
  see also detrusor–sphincter
  dyssynergia
spinal lesions 88
stress incontinence 15, 33–45
  diagnosis and assessment 34
  etiology/risk factors 33–4,
  98
  examination in women 17
  management 35–45, 95
suprapontine lesions 88
surgery
  bladder neck obstruction
  (primary) 62
  bladder outlet obstruction
  60–1
  incontinence 23, 38–42,
  43–5, 95
  overactive bladder 54–5
  PBS/IC 79–80
  urethral stricture 62
  urinary retention following
  95
  vesicovaginal fistula 102

symptoms (lower urinary
  tract)
  history-taking 14–16
  quality of life impact,
  assessment 18
  urodynamic studies 23–4
  UTI 72, 77
  see also specific symptoms

tension-free vaginal tape
  (TVT) 39, 42
terminal dribble 16
tolteradine 51
transitional cell carcinoma,
  cytology 66
transobturator mid-urethral
  sling 39
transrectal digital
  examination of prostate 17,
  58, 59
transrectal ultrasonography
  60
transurethral incision of
  bladder neck and prostate
  61
transurethral resection of
  prostate 60–1
transvaginal electrical
  stimulation 35, 52
tricyclic antidepressants 78,
  84
trospium 51
tumors 64, 65, 69
  malignant *see* malignancy

UK, useful addresses 105–6
ultrasonography 22, 60,
  83
urethra
  bulking agent injection *see*
  bulking agents
  catheterization *see*
  catheterization
  dilatation (treatment) in
  UTI 73
  drug-induced tone
  alterations 97
  functional assessment 28
  incontinence, cause of 31
  sling procedure 38–9
  stricture 57, 62

urethral sphincter, external
  see sphincter
urethral valves, posterior 57,
  58
urge incontinence 15, 32
urgency 15
  in filling cystometry,
  assessment 27
  pregnancy 98
urinalysis
  (laboratory/biochemical
  values) 10–12
  bladder outlet obstruction
  59
  dipstick see dipstick tests
  hematuria 65
  UTI 73
urinary diary see
  frequency/volume chart
urinary incontinence see
  incontinence
urinary retention 95–6, 97,
  99
urinary tract
  anatomy 9
  function 9–13
  infections see infections

urinary tract continued
  symptoms (lower) see
  symptoms and specific
  symptoms
  tumors see tumors
urine
  biochemical tests see
  urinalysis
  cultures see cultures
  cytology, in hematuria 66
  flow 16, 24, 25, 28, 59–60,
  83
  storage see filling
  voiding see voiding
urodynamic studies 23–9
  bladder outlet obstruction
  59–60
  nocturia/nocturnal polyuria
  85
  overactive bladder 47
uroflowmetry 24, 25, 59–60,
  83
urography, intravenous see
  intravenous urography
USA, useful addresses 106
UTI see infections, urinary
  tract

vagina
  estrogen application 75
  fistulous communications
  100–2
  microflora 72
vaginal cones 37, 38
vaginal delivery and stress
  incontinence 33, 98
vaginal tape, tension-free
  (TVT) 39, 42
vesicoureteric reflux 73
vesicovaginal fistula 100–2
voiding (micturition;
  emptying)
  desire, evaluation 26–7
  frequent see frequency
  incomplete 16
  physiology 9–11, 12
  problems with 57–63, 95–6
  symptoms 15–16, 24,
  99–100
voiding cystometry 28

weight loss 48
women see female/women

X-rays see radiography

What the reviewers say:

*a clear, concise, easy to read and beautifully illustrated text.
I am not lending my copy to anyone!*

Professor Stephen R Durham, President, British Society for Allergy & Clinical Immunology,
on *Fast Facts – Rhinitis*, 2nd edn, Sep 2007

*concise, well written and illustrated, colourful, informative and factual…
One to dip in and out of, yet small enough to read cover to cover. Buy
it yourself, but be careful your colleagues don't borrow it indefinitely.*

On *Fast Facts – Asthma*, 2nd edn, in *Primary Health Care*, 2007

*this splendid book shows a lot of originality … an excellent,
well-structured resource for all healthcare professionals*

Mary Baker MBE, Patron, European Parkinson's Disease Association,
on *Fast Facts – Parkinson's Disease*, 2nd edn, Apr 2007

*I strongly recommend this book as a resource for the busy
healthcare professional, both during their training and in practice*

On *Fast Facts – Diseases of the Pancreas and Biliary Tract*,
in *Can J Gastroenterol* 21(3), 2007

*contains very well-constructed tables and boxes which highlight salient
points of diagnosis and management and … a great many tips on how
best to manage patients*

Dr Simon Barton, President, British Association for Sexual Health & HIV,
on *Fast Facts – Sexually Transmitted Infections*, Feb 2007

*… a well-illustrated book that covers the most important ocular
conditions encountered by primary-care physicians*

On *Fast Facts – Ophthalmology*, in Ocular Surgery News, Oct 2006
(Commended, BMA Medical Book Competition, 2007)

www.fastfacts.com

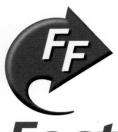

70
key topi
authored b
150 world exper

Fast Facts

the ultimate medical handbook series

- Concise, clear and practical

- Evidence-based and backed up with references

- The perfect balance of text, tables and illustrations

Other urology titles include:

Bladder Cancer 2nd edn

Renal Disorders

Sexually Transmitted Infections 2nd edn

Urinary Stones

New for 2008:

Benign Prostatic Hyperplasia 6th edn

Erectile Dysfunction 4th edn

Fast Facts are for practice, for reference, for teaching and for study.

For a full list visit:
www.fastfacts.com

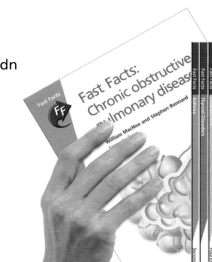